The
Manhattan
Diet

Lose Weight While Living

a Fabulous Life

Eileen Daspin

Quercus

arcus, 33 Baker Street, ... South Wark London ... U 8EW

... on the ... s by John Wiley & ... ons, Inc.

The information contained in this book is not intended to serve as a replacement for professional medical advice. Any use of the information in this book is at the reader's discretion. The author and the publisher specifically disclaim any and all liability arising directly or indirectly from the use or application of any information contained in this book. A health care professional should be consulted regarding your specific situation.

Recipe Credits: p. 222, Tandoori Salmon: Originally published in *Family Circle Eat What You Love and Lose*. All rights reserved; p. 228, Tom Colicchio's Poached Sea Bass with Roasted Tomato Vinaigrette and Fennel Salad: Recipe courtesy of Tom Colicchio; p. 231, Eric Ripert's Grilled Salmon and Herb Salad with Toasted Sesame Seeds and Ponzu Vinaigrette: Recipe courtesy of Eric Ripert; p.232, Pan-Fried Chicken Breasts *Aglio e Olio*: Recipe courtesy of Lidia Bastianich, *Lidia's Family Table* (Knopf, 2004); p. 245, Tomato-Watermelon Salad with Almond Vinaigrette recipe from *New American Table* by Marcus Samuelsson. Copyright © 2009 by Marcus Samuelsson. Reprinted with permission of John Wiley & Sons, Inc.; p. 249, Misticanza: Recipe courtesy of Mario Batali, *Molto Gusto* (Ecco, 2010)

A CIP catalogue record for this book is available from the British Library

ISBN 978 1 78206 168 7

Design by Forty-five Degree Design LLC

Printed and bound in Great Britain by Clays Ltd. St Ives plc.

2 4 6 8 10 9 7 5 3 1

Contents

Introduction

I've been dieting since I was about twelve years old. That year, at five feet seven, I tipped the scale at about eight stone and survived on a diet of homemade gelatine concocted from low-cal fizzy drinks and gelatine powder, low-fat cottage cheese mixed with Sweet'N Low and cinnamon (to taste like the filling from a Danish pastry), frozen prawns, and iceberg lettuce doused in low-cal Thousand Island dressing.

As I got older, I expanded my horizons. I did the grapefruit diet, I fasted, and I tried Weight Watchers. For a while, I even went to a therapist. I lost weight and I gained it. And I lost it.

It's been years since I followed an actual weight-loss diet, but the yo-yo mentality stuck with me like a bad pop song. I'm never not dieting. It's part of who I am.

I got the idea for *The Manhattan Diet* in the summer of 2009 after reading a story in the *New York Times* comparing the overweight and obesity rates of the five boroughs that make up

New York City: Queens, Brooklyn, the Bronx, Staten Island, and Manhattan. According to the article, which drew on research from the Centers for Disease Control, Manhattan was not only the thinnest borough, it was the skinniest of all sixty-two counties in New York State.

Given my backstory, the piece was one of those things that just resonated. In spite of everything—the four-star restaurants, street food culture, chefmania, snack shops galore, Dylan's Candy Bar and its many imitators—Manhattanites, and Manhattan women in particular, were svelte.

The idea for a book unspooled in five minutes. If Manhattan women had figured out how to keep fighting trim in this punishingly foodie environment, there must be something to learn from them. I had a million questions: How do Manhattan Dieters think about food? What do they eat? What don't they eat? What and how do they order in restaurants? Do they cook? Do they order in? Are they thin just because they walk a lot? Where do they shop? Are their habits different from the rest of the country's?

I set out to uncover just what the Manhattan Diet is and how the rules here can be adopted by women in Orlando, Florida, where I grew up; or Milton, Massachusetts, my mom's hometown; or Three Rivers, California, where my friend Chris lives. In other words, how could the lessons of Manhattan eating apply to places that weren't Manhattan?

To find out, I started talking to every thin, fit, stylish woman around me. I debriefed diet and exercise pros, psychologists, academics, chefs, and waiters. I reviewed studies and haunted the aisles of Whole Foods. I visited gyms and restaurants and took yoga seminars, Spin classes, and even pole-dancing lessons. I was the George Plimpton of the diet set.

A year later I had finished my interviews, assembled my data, collected recipes and tips, and broken bread with everyone from *Food & Wine* editor Dana Cowin to celebrity Spin instructor Stacey Griffith to glam fitness buff Cristina Cuomo. I conducted my own research, studying the diets of a select group of Manhattan svelties, and I compiled it all here, in *The Manhattan Diet*.

The feeding and exercise habits of my co-denizens, it turns out, are an artful weave of the best diet practices on the planet. The speed version goes something like this: Eat well, but not too much. Walk like a maniac. Cook at home. Leave a little something on the plate. Indulge your sweet tooth. Don't go hungry. Don't deprive yourself. Eat whole foods; dump anything with *diet* in the name. Water is good. A glass of wine is fine, too, if you like. Toss the Lean Cuisine. Eat your vegetables.

The unabridged narrative is a little more counterintuitive. With every interview, I uncovered something unexpected. Fat, for example, is a staple here. Manhattan loves its butter, extra-virgin olive oil, triple-cream cheeses, whole milk, cashews, and almonds. It is a town that embraces "buttery flavour spreads," skimmed milk, and reduced-fat string cheese selectively, as in when no one else is watching. This is as much about aesthetics as it is a point of pride. Manhattan Dieters don't think of themselves as fatties; therefore, they don't eat like dieters.

It's a similar story for carbs. Apologies to Doctors Arthur Agatston, Robert Atkins, and Pierre Dukan and other carbophobes, but Manhattan Dieters love their pasta, their risotto, and their bagels. This is not what I expected when I asked twenty-five women to keep diet diaries for me. Given how demonized carbs have become in the last decade, I expected to see mostly red meat, chicken, fish, and vegetables. Instead, my ladies were mainlining grain products. On some intuitive level, Manhattan Dieters have concluded that the anti-carb faction is just wrong. They've tried it and discovered it's not for them.

That to me is the beauty of the Manhattan Diet. It is based on the real-life experience of real people—millions of them—over many decades. As far as I can tell, if there is a difference between the average Manhattanite and the average dieter anywhere else, it comes down to attitude: Manhattan Dieters aren't afraid of food.

They love it, the way Europeans do. Eating is entertainment; it's fun, healthy, and necessary. What on the surface might seem like stumbling blocks—the restaurants, the gourmet markets, the chefs, the foodie obsessions—instead underscore how much food is loved here. And that makes all the difference. Manhattan Dieters are eaters. They're also big home cooks and food and ingredient snobs. And they're surrounded by people who think the same way.

It's hard to dissect the influences and the roots. Are Manhattan Dieters thin and fashionable because they're surrounded by other thin and fashionable types? Are they svelte because they eat well, or does being svelte make them watch their waistlines?

It's all of the above, and, of course, more. The Manhattan Diet is a state of mind—it's practical, and its lessons are transferable. Read on to learn them.

1

Forget the French
How We Act

I am obsessed with food—on about twenty different levels. I get near-erotic thrills from beautiful produce. I read recipes for fun. I worry about what my ten-year-old daughter eats and track the comings and goings of chefs and the openings and closings of restaurants. I'm a leafy greens, wholegrains freak. I grew up in a home where my mom made stuff from scratch, even bagels, ice cream, bucatini all'amatriciana. I've been on a diet since I was about twelve and can ballpark the calories of pretty much anything, with maybe a 5 percent margin of error. To top it off, I'm married to a chef. It's quite the cocktail.

I'm lucky to live in a place where I am surrounded by people who are obsessed with food. That place is Manhattan, which I think of as me multiplied by 1.6 million. We all have wildly different life stories: moms who cooked, moms who didn't; fat when we were kids, skinny when we were kids. We're meat eaters or not, reflexive dieters or caution-to-the-wind types.

We worry about eating too much, about not being able to eat enough, and about not being able to stop eating. It is a tangled love–hate dynamic complicated by an unhealthy interest in celebrity chefs, imported gelato, bad street food, and anything to do with restaurateur Danny Meyer. Have you eaten at Maialino? Lincoln? Eataly? Colicchio & Sons? (Fill in the blank with any new restaurant, grocery, bar, or gelateria.)

I have to be honest. Sometimes it's exhausting: not just keeping up with the endless trends—bee pollen, artisanal popcorn, Momofuku spin-offs—but deconstructing every single morsel that we eat or consider eating. I'd like to take a break. But I'm obsessed, so I can't.

We even have a neurotic foodie mayor, the billionaire Michael Bloomberg, who is in his late sixties. Mayor Mike worries so much about his appearance that he maintains a running weight-loss competition with one of his friends. An unflattering photo in the press is said to tip him into weeks of soul-searching and cranky dieting. As mayor, Bloomberg has led the charge for a city-wide ban on trans fats, has forced chain restaurants to post calorie counts, has tried to shame chefs into cutting the amount of salt in dishes, and has campaigned against sugary beverages. Yet the man who got the city to cut back on smoking cigarettes apparently can't wean himself from peanut butter and burnt-bacon sandwiches and super-salty bagels.

He is hardly alone. Nearly everyone I know suffers from a variation on the foodie disorder. We're control freaks. We clearly spend too much psychic energy and way too much disposable income on food-driven pursuits. We live and breathe what I think of as the Manhattan mystery, which is this: we are obsessed with food, yet the city's twenty-thousand restaurants, four-star chefs, candy shops, doughnut carts, and endless other temptations don't show up on our thighs, butts, or other visible body parts.

Studies do show that 42 percent of the city is overweight or obese. But that's way better than the nation as a whole (in which 67 percent of the population is overweight or obese) and, believe it or not, *way* better than Colorado (57.6 percent), which usually places first in the publicity-generating surveys of the skinniest and the fattest states. In fact, if you look at the 2010 combined obesity and overweight statistics, the borough of Manhattan is thinner than every state in the country—by 13.6 percentage points.

All of this raises the following questions: Is there something about living here that allows Manhattanites to indulge in every cuisine, sneak in junk food, eat out more often than seems mathematically possible, and yet somehow keep our girlish (and boyish) figures? Have Manhattanites unwittingly stumbled upon the eater's holy grail? The diet that isn't a diet? The diet that actually works?

On the face of it, this idea might sound silly. How can an accident of geography produce the answer to the ten pounds we've all been trying to shed since before the Weight Watchers era? Up until recently, the prospect never occurred to me, and I've been keeping tabs on the eating habits of Manhattanites since the 1980s. I wrote

. . . .

How They Diet

SARAH JESSICA PARKER

She claims to eat everything from lamb shanks to bagels with cream cheese, but she has also helped popularize the BluePrintCleanse and has been photographed sipping from one of the company's baby bottle–shaped containers. The diet includes six juices a day, which add up to between 1,000 and 1,200 calories daily.

. . . .

about food and restaurants for the *Wall Street Journal* for years and am married to the restaurant world through my husband, the chef Cesare Casella. I've written cookbooks with him, and as his wife I get invited to some pretty swank foodie events: restaurant openings, wine tastings, private dinners, and weekends in Connecticut where everyone pitches in, Big Chill-style, except that the cooks in the kitchen are Cesare, Daniel Boulud, and Dorothy Hamilton, the owner of the International Culinary Center in Manhattan.

All of my friends are relatively thin. And yes, we all exercise. We share grocery strategies. Yet we live in diners. We rush to beat one another with reservations at new restaurants. We drink alcohol. We eat a lot of dark chocolate—and pizza. Yet it never occurred to me until I decided to write this book that just as French women don't get fat, neither do the ladies of Manhattan.

Forget the damn French. Manhattan women are clearly on to something. Love New York or hate it, there is something to be learned from this borough's geography, eating habits, attitudes, neuroses, and frozen yogurt consumption. Whatever that secret might be—and I will discuss the options in this book—it has produced a tribe full of size 2 (UK 6), 4 (UK 8), and 6 (UK 10) yoga moms and executives-cum-marathoners, not to mention women like me (UK size 14) who are just in better shape than we have a right to be, given our surroundings.

One-third of all the people I know are not fat, let alone obese. Sure, some would like to lose 10 or 15 pounds, but if I had to guesstimate the obesity rate in my social circle, it would be maybe 3 percent, about the same as Japan's. Without overstating my case, I can prove myself right by just sticking to the postcodes and neighbourhoods that make up what I tend to think of as Manhattan: meaning the Upper East and Upper West Sides, the land of the Gossip Girls and "social X-rays."

This Manhattan is even skinnier than France, where 14 percent of adults are obese. On the Upper East Side, where Mayor Bloomberg lives, the obesity rate is about 8 percent—the same as it is on the Upper West Side, where I live, and even in the West Village, where the citizens of postcode 10011 are surrounded by thirty pizzerias, ten Starbucks, and twenty different supermarkets. In a land where you can never be too rich or too thin, Manhattanites, it turns out, are often both.

You're probably thinking, "Ha! Manhattan is full of *Dirty Sexy Money* types who've got nothing better to do than double up on morning Spin classes so they can burn one thousand calories before lunch." And you're right. One reason there are so many skinnies and so many healthies in Manhattan is that people who live in the postcodes of my world have money, and often a lot of it. On the Upper East Side, the per capita income is more than $120,000 (£70,000), making it one of the densest concentrations of wealth in the country.

You can't turn the page of a magazine or click through a gossip site without learning that Gwyneth Paltrow works out with trainer Tracy Anderson, is a patient of detox doctor Alejandro Junger, and lives on vegan fare, meal-replacement shakes ($350/£215 for a twenty-one-day supply), and kale. Julianne Moore works with trainer David Kirsch, does yoga, and prefers granola bars, yogurt, and breakfast cereal. Celebrity publicist Peggy Siegal is attended to by so many health and beauty experts that she handed out a list of their names as a party favour to the guests at her sixtieth birthday bash.

Granted, in these circles, cost is no bother. And that means a lot when you're talking about four-star restaurants, organic free-range eggs, personal trainers, private chefs, nutritionists, and the dubious luxury of seven-day juice cleanses delivered to your doorstep by stylishly attired messengers.

But having lived here for thirty years, I know it's not *all* about having money. Really. When I walk to the grocery store, there are a few key things going on. For instance, note the verb *walk*. I walk to the grocery store, then I walk home from the grocery store with about nine kilos of purchases in two bags. I do that two or three times a week. Everyone here walks to the supermarket, to the kids' school, to the dentist, or to the corner newsstand to pick up a newspaper, a magazine, or a lottery ticket. You get the idea.

Paula Seefeldt is a health counsellor in New York. Recently she worked with a client who had moved from Manhattan to San Francisco and put on two stone in the process. Both counsellor and patient strapped on pedometers for a few days, and when they compared numbers, Seefeldt was registering 9,000 to 15,000 steps daily. Her client tallied 3,000. How to start the Manhattan Diet? Try a pair of trainers.

Let's go back to my supermarket visit for a minute. The trip is about a ten- to twelve-minute walk from my apartment. As long as it's not the dead of winter, when everyone is bundled up in down coats and mufflers, I am using that time to take note of the people around me on the sidewalk: the bare midriffs, the tone of the upper arms, the quality of the handbags. It's second nature here. We constantly compare ourselves to everyone around us. How do we measure up? Do we look younger, older, more rested, more successful? Do we have better taste, better abs? I will often stop a woman on the street and ask her where she purchased some item of clothing she is wearing or tell her she looks great, because she does. I'm not hitting on her; I'm being appreciative.

I grew up in Orlando, Florida. Today, if I walk around the suburb there where my dad lives, I'm alone except for maybe a gardener. If by chance there *is* someone on the street, he is usually in sweatpants, not dressed up to show off for other pedestrians.

On my way to buy groceries in Manhattan, I pass Barneys Co-Op, a speciality clothing store; Stuart Weitzman, an upscale shoe shop; and Loehmann's, which sells discount designer wear. The windows are filled with mannequins and images of toned and fit models, limbs akimbo, in some funky outfit that is appropriate only on a person with a body mass index of 17.5 or less. As I walk, my internal style monitor clicks on, capturing how everyone around me looks, calculating how I measure up, and logging those comparisons inside my brain.

What does all of this have to do with the Manhattan Diet? Just about everything. If all of your pals are doing yoga and Pilates and running in the park three times a week, chances are you will start doing the same. The famous "Do My Friends Make Me Look Fat?" study done by Harvard researchers found that having obese friends makes it more likely that you too will be obese. Living in Manhattan creates the opposite effect. We are surrounded by slim and fit colleagues, friends, shop assistants, and strangers on the train, and we feel pressured to look like them. Manhattan is one giant peer pressure cooker.

When I moved to Manhattan after college in 1980, I was twenty-one years old, five feet seven, and nearly twelve stone. I didn't exercise regularly (or at all, actually), and on occasion I would buy logs of chocolate chip cookie dough—not to bake, but to eat raw, slice by slice. My eating habits were awful. I inhaled Brie by the pound and made salad dressing from mayonnaise and ketchup.

Thirty years later, my weight fluctuates between ten and ten-and-a-half stone. I eat at my husband's restaurant once a week—my favourite dish is made with pancetta, scrambled eggs, and mixed salad leaves—and I bring home mortadella and aged Parmigiano-Reggiano for snacks. I roast kale and steam mussels. I do yoga and also jog and walk two to three miles a day.

I still have a spoonful or two of cookie dough when I'm baking with my daughter, but I'm no longer the fat girl I once was. What happened? I'm not a nutritionist, a psychiatrist, or any sort of medical researcher with multiple degrees. I'm a journalist who watches what goes on around me. What happened to me in the last thirty years? I became a Manhattan Dieter.

Now, I'm the first to say that the way I eat, exercise, order in restaurants, and shop for groceries is not so interesting. But if you combine me with a hundred other women who are just as focused, just as obsessed, and just as committed to being healthy, it starts to add up to something. And that's what the Manhattan Diet is: anecdotal and true to life. It is an examination of my world and the people in it: my friends, my networks, my friends' networks, and their networks' networks. It is the collective wisdom of a small group of women who like to eat, who deal with temptation, and who somehow manage to keep fit in spite of being moms, wives, single, stressed out at work, or stressed out at home—in other words, women who live with the same pressures as women everywhere, with the difference of having figured out a daily diet that works with their lives.

All Manhattanites aren't angels. When I was writing this book, I met too many women who keep trim with regimens that I just don't believe in. Some of my subjects eat way too many energy bars, drink way too many health shakes, and take way too many supplements instead of eating whole foods. They scrub out their digestive tracts with cleanses and produce very expensive urine with juice fasts. But I can't ignore those things, because they are part of the Manhattan Diet, so you will read about them in chapter 8.

Manhattan women eat candy and chew gum—a lot of candy and gum. But it's okay, because they also consume a lot of romaine lettuce, carrots, broccoli, brown rice, and wild salmon. You can read about that balance and the importance of not feeling deprived in chapter 3. You'll also learn the exercise secrets of busy New Yorkers, how we order in restaurants, and what we've learned from working with experts.

The Manhattan Diet is not a by-the-numbers prescription to health but rather a report from the dieting front lines with universal lessons. Every woman who reads this book will identify with the characters in it, because they will be like her. The women are real and have something to say and something to share. The bottom line is that you don't have to live in Manhattan to eat, exercise, shop for groceries, or cook like a Manhattanite. We do that for you. So lose weight and enjoy!

2

A Manhattan State of Mind

How We Think

In Manhattan, size matters, and in ways you might not have thought about. There are more than 1.6 million people living here, on a sliver of land smaller than Walmart's total retail space. That makes Manhattan the most densely populated piece of land in the United States. Manhattanites have to have tiny appliances to fit in their tiny kitchens, which are size-appropriate for their teensy-weensy apartments. They have miniature dogs and equally miniature furniture.

Apartment life is cramped, and that is where I begin: with the fact that Manhattanites are thin and fit, at least in part because of circumstances. More people want to live here than there's room for. City apartments are insanely expensive and equally claustrophobic. The apartment I live in with my husband and my daughter is twelve hundred square feet, the average size for the city. It's in a lovely pre-World War II building on a tree-lined street next to a park and has two bedrooms, each about twelve by twelve feet. Before this, the three of us lived in a one-bedroom apartment that was even smaller, and before that, when I was single, I lived in a fourteen-by-fourteen-foot studio with a kitchenette, a foldout bed, and a dining table that I kept collapsed behind a desk. Our current kitchen is just ten feet by three feet. There's no island, no double-wide refrigerator, no espresso machine. I store soda water under our CD player in the living room because we don't have a pantry.

But lucky me! It turns out that my space, or the lack of it, prompts me to behave better, at least from a health point of view. Because my kitchen is small, I shop for groceries three, four, or five times a week. It's a time suck and means that my grocery bills are ridiculously high. But my produce, meats, and dairy products are super-fresh, and I'm forced to buy packaged foods in apartment-sized doses.

Apparently that's key, because smaller containers lead to eating less, according to Brian Wansink, a professor at Cornell University. Wansink has done hundreds of studies examining the ways that people eat, and his book, *Mindless Eating*, is something of a bible among Manhattan's nutrition set. The studies are often hilarious and usually very telling. My favourite is the soup bowl he rigged up to refill until the unsuspecting diner declared that she'd eaten enough. It took a lot of soup.

Wansink believes that packaging is particularly influential, because the size of a box or container subtly suggests the right amount to consume. When you've got more of something on hand, you tend to eat more of it, whether it's M&M's, spaghetti, or celery hearts. Wansink and his colleagues tested forty-seven products. Each time the result was the same. Plant food, cereal, laundry detergent—it didn't matter. Hefty sizing triggered hefty consumption. Conclusion for Manhattanites: lacking roomy kitchen storage, they eat less.

I can totally vouch for this theory. My cabinets just can't accommodate suburban family packs and tubs-o'-whatever, so I buy the 500-gram bag of porridge oats, not the one-kilogram one. I buy maple syrup by height (seven inches max), and other wee things: the one-kilo box of sugar, the 225-gram jar of peanut butter, and single-serve containers of yogurt. If I eat half a carton of Rocky Road ice cream when the container is half a litre, I think, Eek! half a litre. But it's better than a litre, which is where I might have stopped had I purchased a big tub.

It's no surprise that I'm always running out of something and dashing out for milk, eggs, or butter. When I go out, I see a lot of people just like me: neighbours who've popped out for some coffee filters, strangers lined up at the newsstand, window shoppers, whatever. Part of this is functional—people are actually buying what they need. But the crowded sidewalks are also another example of how small apartments affect behaviour. Who wants to be stuck in a twelve-hundred-square-foot box all day long? Not me, and not all the other folks I run into when I'm out and about. It's one of those unintended consequences of city life.

To escape desirable but claustrophobic apartments, Manhattanites try to get out as much as possible, whether it's for dinner, to run an errand, or just for fresh air. By definition, they have to walk or take public transportation to their destination, since only a quarter of us own cars. One-fifth of Manhattanites walk to work. And when they're doing all that walking, they're not standing in front of an open refrigerator deciding what to eat, they're not planted in front of their flat-screen TV, and they're not on Facebook connecting with lost high school friends. They're burning calories and strengthening muscles. Meanwhile, because everyone else is out doing the same thing, no one ever knows whom they might run into. So people try to look good. When they go to Starbucks for a latte, it's usually not in sweats and a ratty

T-shirt; it's in form-fitting jeans, a smart-looking jacket, and lipstick.

As human behaviour goes, this is all pretty standard. People are influenced by their surroundings, whether they know it or not. I want to look like the other women around me. Walking up Madison Avenue, I can't help but look at all the skinny, beautiful, fit people and feel the tug.

"What's your apartment like versus mine? What's your outfit like versus mine? What's your body like versus mine? We don't know it consciously, but we are always comparing," says Patricia Duffy, fifty-five. I've known Patricia for about fifteen years. She used to work in the restaurant division of American Express and circled the globe eating and drinking in amazing places. Her travels eventually led her to Cesare, whose family had a Michelin-starred restaurant in Lucca, and once Cesare and I became a couple, to me.

Patricia is a dear friend, and we have spent countless evenings and weekends together with our families—at the loft she and her husband renovated here in the city, at the farmhouse they own in upstate New York, and at the old olive press they have converted into a beautiful home in the hills of Tuscany. This morning we are drinking black tea at a Scandinavian café on the corner of Central Park South and 58th Street and talking about the subtle and overt ways Manhattan affects how we think about our bodies.

"Statistics might not bear me out, but in other cities, you can't sit at a café and see a parade of people who look like they came out of Condé Nast," she says, referring to the magazine company that publishes *Vogue* and *Vanity Fair*. "In this city, we are mobile. We sit at counters and watch people. In Minneapolis, I'd pull on my sweats and get in the car. Here, people are out walking and looking at other people. The minute you get to an airport outside New York, the people in sweat clothes look like they haven't sweated in a really long time."

. . . .

How They Diet

TINA FEY

When the *30 Rock* star was twenty-nine, she lost about two and a half pounds with Weight Watchers. That's when she learned how to eat properly. Before that, Fey has said, she used to go all day without eating, then start snacking on cake and finish the day at McDonald's.

. . . .

Patricia is the quintessential Manhattan Dieter. She is slim, petite, passionate and informed about food and wine, but she watches what she eats like the Little Red Hen counting her grains of wheat. If she overindulges one evening, she's in the gym early the next morning working it off. Yet the Patricia who is my friend today is a very different woman from the one in sweats who moved here in 1986 from Minneapolis. For starters, she's about two clothing sizes smaller. She is also now a part-time stay-at-home mom and an exercise nut. But more important, by living here she's learned to feed herself in a way that she says was impossible growing up. Back in Wisconsin, where she was born, Patricia remembers all-you-can-eat Friday fish fries, oversized portions, and the understanding that you cleared your plate before you got up from the table.

The guiding principle was quantity. A good meal was a big meal. When she travelled, she brought her fat trousers so she could eat even more. That started to change after she began travelling to Europe. She remembers in particular a two-and-a-half-week trip to Italy with John, her husband. They ate and drank whatever they wanted and had pasta at every meal, but when they got home, Patricia found that her trousers were loose. It was a total eye-opener, she says. "We were having small portions—nothing was smothered with sauce—and a small salad and wine. Plus, we were moving around a lot." Over time, that eating style became her own.

I love going out to eat with Patricia, because she's always the one to order something fattening that I want to taste but don't have the nerve to get myself. She actually reads the menu for something that appeals to her, not just something healthy, so that her meal is pleasurable and she can linger over the tastes and flavours. She is especially interested in things she can't or wouldn't make at home, and she would no sooner order grilled lamb chops or roasted chicken than fried mozzarella sticks topped with melted American cheese and shoved between two slices of bread—an item I actually saw on a Denny's menu recently.

She is, however, pretty vigilant about portion control, and instead of an appetizer, a main course, and dessert, she orders two appetizers. When she cooks at home, she applies the same principles. She is fantastic in front of a stove and loves to entertain, throwing big dinner parties for which she'll roast a rack of lamb and serve it with rosemary potatoes, sautéed spinach, and a tower of homemade focaccia. Or she will throw together orecchiette, with sausage, broccoli, and heaps of Parmigiano-Reggiano cheese. There are always multiple bottles of wine, including the Sauvignon Blanc made from the vineyard she and John own in Italy.

There is no concession to weight watching. It's all about hearty filling food and eating enough so you're not full, just undersatiated. It's been years since Patricia even owned fat trousers, so her approach clearly works. "The stress of gaining one and a half stone just makes you want to stay away from too much food," she says.

Not every place on the map puts a premium on looks. But Manhattan is headquarters to some of the biggest image industries. There's beauty, from niche brands like Bobbi Brown and MAC to big Revlon-style firms. There's fashion, both retail and the design end. There's also advertising, media, publishing, and so on. And the people who work in those businesses go to work dressed for the job. I don't mean *dressed* as in putting on clothes. I mean dressed *up*.

Spend half an hour in the lobby of the Condé Nast building around ten in the morning—or at any time, actually—and you will see what I am talking about. Dozens of tall, willowy women in their twenties and thirties will stream through the revolving doors in an astounding array of costume jewellery, headgear, things that wrap around their waists, and capes. They'll be in skinny trousers and Chanel jackets, carrying totes and handbags that cost what we spend to put our daughter through a year of private school. Their look is gravity defying, lifting them above mere mortals. These women walk around the office in their Christian Louboutin heels all day long. Don't ask me how.

And they're not alone. At any given hour, similar displays are unfolding all over town—in the tower where L'Oreal America is located, at ad agencies like Porter/Novelli or Ogilvy and Mather, in the lobby of Warner Music, and at the offices of Calvin Klein and Donna Karan. Regardless of the particular style of clothing, people dress up. Every city, of course, has its dress code—I think of the abs and pecs and glutes on parade in Los Angeles, the studied casual combo of perfectly faded jeans and Jack Purcell trainers. The point is, Manhattan is more formal than many U.S. cities, closer to a European aesthetic than a Californian one. Like the way travellers used to dress up to take a plane or a train in the 1960s and 1970s, people here dress to be in public. It is both a form of showing off and a throwback to a more elegant time.

The emphasis on looks affects how Manhattanites size one another up and how they think about themselves. "People want to be with people who reflect how they want to be," says Pam Liebman, CEO of the Corcoran Group, one of the largest estate agencies in the country. "When you want to be successful in business, it doesn't hurt to look good. As shallow as it may be, I think that people look at you and think if you take care of yourself, you will take care of them, too."

Liebman is forty-seven and has been running the company since 2001, when she was named to replace founder Barbara

Corcoran, who was stepping aside. Liebman is what my dad would describe as a dynamo—peppy, intense, upbeat, a go-getter—and it's easy to see how she landed at the top of a $4.2 billion (£2.6 billion) estate agency. I first interviewed Liebman about ten years ago when I did a story about CEOs and their diets for the *Wall Street Journal*. I remembered how chatty she'd been about the topic, so I when I started researching for this book, I called her to see if we could meet.

Liebman graciously invited me to Fred's, the restaurant inside Barneys, the baroquely trendy Madison Avenue speciality store. Fred's is sleek and polished and full of women who have the means to order whatever they want but who tend to pick at salads. When we arrived, the restaurant staff was both deferential and discreet, treating Liebman as one of those people who don't have to ask for anything; the thing just materializes. After we were escorted to Liebman's regular table, a waiter brought out iced tea without any prompting, and the chef, Mark Strausman, slid over to pay his compliments.

Liebman is tiny—five feet one and a half, about seven and a half stone—blonde, and kind of a diet maniac, but in a good way. Over lunch, I remember why I wanted to talk to her in the first place. She is up on all kinds of exercise trends, food crazes, restaurant openings, and health news. She can toggle easily between the benefits of the Alkaline Diet (something to do with food-combining and burning fat) to Tanya Zuckerbrot, a Manhattan diet star who keeps her clients on a regimen of high-fibre crackers. She herself has done the Isogenix cleanse ("I think it's good to detox"), and she hears good things about BluePrintCleanse, a trendy juice fast.

By five o'clock each morning, Liebman says, her fitness brain is already switched on. That's the time she starts her Insanity Workout, a DVD programme she bought at the suggestion of a friend who is a professional football player. The regimen is an hour long and involves a gruelling series of push-ups, jumps, and other moves that leave me exhausted just hearing about them.

Before doing the Insanity Workout, Liebman was popping in a similar DVD for a programme called P9OX Extreme Home Fitness. For a taste of what "Extreme Fitness" means, check out the company's cable-television infomercials. They are intense. I couldn't see Liebman's biceps or abs at our lunch because she was wearing a long-sleeved silk blouse. But I imagine they look not unlike those of the women in the Insanity Workout video—that is, extremely firm.

Liebman says she thinks about her diet every day, not in the sense of satisfying her nutritional needs, but for how her diet translates into her world. She thinks about how she looks and the impression she makes on others, the way she looks on television, what restaurants are new, what the food trends are, whether her staff is eating properly, and whether her exercise regimen is challenging enough or is getting stale. It is nonstop and all-encompassing.

When Liebman was looking for a motivational speaker to address her sales staff at a recent meeting, she reached out not to a property tycoon like Donald Trump but to Danny Meyer, the foodie guru who built one hipster restaurant—Union Square Café—into a mini empire. She helped get Weight Watchers classes for her staff in the office and gave a stair-climbing machine to an assistant as a birthday present after the staffer mentioned that she didn't have time to go to a gym to work out.

Liebman says her approach to eating is balanced. She listens to her body and works hard not to get hungry. She never skips breakfast. She reads food labels carefully—so much so that her kids won't go grocery shopping with her—and keeps her desk stocked with snacks like protein bars and nuts. Her meals are moderate, mostly simple grilled items with no heavy sauces, and she drinks two litres of water every day. "My friends say, 'Oh, you're not eating.' But I don't think of myself as dieting. If I feel like having dessert, I'll have it. If not, I'll skip it."

There is no way, of course, to shoehorn the eating and exercising habits of so many people into one neat little box. There are as many ways of thinking about food in Manhattan as there are bodies, and Pam Liebman and Patricia Duffy are two very different examples. If you interviewed a hundred more women, you would probably get another hundred takes on what a good diet is. The single common thread I've been able to discern in my subjects is the amount of time they spend *thinking* about eating.

The process is constant. It is unrelenting. It is detailed. It's researched and data driven. And it's full of conviction. The right way is organic. The right way is portion control. The right way is low-carb, low-fat, small snacks throughout the day, and three square meals. For every woman who embraces calorie counting, there are just as many who have simply sworn off cheese or who eat the same thing every day as a hedge against temptation or as a concession to habit.

. . . .

What the Butler Saw

Chris Ely was the longtime butler for Brooke Astor, the now-deceased socialite and widow of Vincent Astor, the great-great grandson of America's first multimillionaire, John Jacob Astor. Ely has also worked for a variety of other Manhattan clients and is now dean of the Household Management Institute at the International Culinary Center in Manhattan. I interviewed him for his insight.

What is it about the people you've worked for? How do they, in the words of the Duchess of Windsor, stay rich and thin?

From twenty years ago, the difference is they aren't hitting the butter, they're not hitting the alcohol, they're not eating cholesterol. If you notice, the Upper East Side isn't dotted with McDonald's. People eat at home a lot, or they go to restaurants and get grilled fish. To them, fats are bad, carbohydrates are bad. They will have three lettuce leaves for lunch and move on. They push food around on their plates. They can have as much as they want and when they want it, but they don't.

Is it health driven? Vanity? What's the worry?

A lot of people have very expensive wardrobes. The last thing they want is to put on an ounce or go up a clothing size. We're talking about hundreds of thousands of dollars. Starving themselves is a way of life. They're on a permanent diet. It's not healthy.

Do they do anything right?

They have the best medical care in the world. Many of them watch the same newscasts, read the same newspapers and magazines. They can be a little hyper about these things. They are looking to live longer. All of a sudden there is a new threat—say, diabetes. They go into the kitchen and make you get rid of anything with high-fructose corn syrup in it. It's hard for a personal chef. What do you do with an employer who is screaming at you because they don't want to get fat?

So what do they eat?

Lots of chicken breast, salads, fresh vegetables, that sort of thing. They will also have a plain piece of grilled fish. Most avoid red meat. Pork is out of the question. Dessert would be fruit. For dinner, it might be a mozzarella and tomato salad, maybe a courgette or other squash soup. Nothing with cream in it. There would be fresh vegetables or a puree. If you have someone who needs iron, there might be spinach. You are always trained to resist the butter and refined flour. And carbs.

What about breakfast and snacks?

A lot don't have any breakfast. Their refrigerators are like Starbucks, with three types of milk: full fat, no fat, lactose-free.

For snacks there are some strange choices: rice cakes with
artificial sweetener on top, toast sprayed with olive oil.

**Mrs. Astor was a famous hostess. What sorts of things
would she serve?**

Mrs. Astor would tailor her lunch to who was coming. You're
not going to serve a barbecue to the ladies who lunch. If you
also have kids at the table, at least give them a little macaroni and cheese. The adults like it, too, and take a little bite.

. . . .

I am just as guilty as my subjects. The other night, Cesare
and I went to Bedford, New York, to celebrate our tenth anniver-
sary. I wanted to check out the Bedford Post Inn, the Relais &
Châteaux franchise that Richard Gere and his wife, Carey Low-
ell, had opened there; it is known for both its food and its yoga
barn. I ate very little during the day so I could have a big dinner.
I know that's not good, and it just leaves me really hungry at dinner time, but that's me. We sat down—next to George Stepha-
nopoulos—and the usual cascade of doubts and worries set in. I
have to have fish because it's the least fattening. But how is it
prepared? Skip over the pasta choices—a total no-no, although
the squash ravioli sounds tempting—they remind me of when I
lived in Italy and went skiing with my friend Lisa. I don't really
want chicken. How many appetizers should I get?

All of this ran through my head in less than two minutes. In the
end, I chose mushrooms in a broth, a skate dish, and a side of
Brussels sprouts with spicy walnuts. When the waiter gave us
bread, I ate three pieces in spite of trying to stop myself. Then,
because the chef recognized Cesare, the complimentary dishes
starting arriving: squash soup. Mozzarella and anchovies. I ate all
that, too, with great guilt. Then there were pumpkin ice cream
sandwiches for dessert. Had I not been possessed with dieting

angst, I would have eaten two small satisfying meals earlier in the day, ordered what I wanted at dinner, and not inhaled everything in sight, including the CD-sized chocolate chip cookie that was left on my pillow in our room.

But possessed I am. Variations on that inner dialogue spin through the heads of almost all of the women I know, multiple times a day. I'm not saying it's good, I'm just saying it's probably more the rule than the exception.

I've known Nancy Farkas for about seven years. Our daughters have been friends since they were two and three, and we've become close as the girls have grown up. Nancy is smart, accomplished, and great-looking. She's got a very matter-of-fact New York way about her, and I admire her just-get-it-done attitude. She's a lawyer for a large bank and strikes me as incredibly competent, no-nonsense. I would not want to be on the other side of the negotiating table from her. But when it comes to food, I'd say that she's as unbalanced as I am.

"I think about every single thing that I put in my mouth before I put it in my mouth," is how she starts our conversation. We are sitting on the beach on Long Island, and our daughters are playing in the sand a few yards away. We're both glad the girls are out of earshot, because one constant worry among Manhattan women is that they will pass on their food issues to their daughters. In my opinion, Nancy always looks fit, but she's often on a diet in which she eats only milk and vegetables on alternating days. When she's not on that diet, she seems to me to eat pretty well, although I'm now hearing about her secret monologue for the first time. It sounds an awful lot like my Bedford Post Inn soliloquy.

"There has to be a rationalization behind [what I'm eating], as a reward for some injustice, in support of the diet of the day," she tells me. "I've taken mindful eating beyond all levels of rationality. Every morsel has a story attached to it. I get up and make my latte; I decide if it is going to be skinny latte or regular latte or iced black coffee. The decision turns on the diet I am following that day. If I lived in Kansas, it just wouldn't be the same. The emphasis wouldn't be there."

Some of what motivates her is environmental. Nancy works on Wall Street and says the women around her are either very young and very attractive or very old and very unattractive. Going to the office each day magnifies the feeling she has of being caught in the middle of those groups. What's more, she feels assaulted by eating opportunities. Everywhere she looks, there is the chance to eat, whether it is something good or something bad. In those circumstances, she has trained herself to say no to everything.

She wishes she could turn off the commentary, but she can't. "There are bigger problems in the world I could be thinking about. It would be so simple if I picked a path and stuck to it and lost ten pounds. I could free up all the mental energy to do other things."

As I said, Nancy and I are good friends, so I think she was more open with me than some of the other women I spoke to were. On some level it's just not cool to acknowledge how crazy you are about food. More often than not, I felt I was up against food bravado: women who claimed to be secure in their diets, who said they didn't think or worry about food, who just ate what they wanted. But when I asked these women, dozens of them, to keep food diaries, their carefree I-eat-what-I-want attitude disappeared.

At least half of the women asked how their diaries compared to other women's. Almost everyone worried that she was eating too much or eating the wrong things at the wrong times of the day. Many mentioned that they ate better while keeping the diary because they didn't want to have to write down the bad bits for me to see. A few gave up two or three days into the exercise because they found it too trying. One friend told me she lost her diary. Another kept saying I was going to be shocked at the quantities she consumed. Then there were the questions: if I have digestive biscuits at two in the morning, does that count for Monday or Tuesday? Can I start tomorrow? I just had a piece of pizza. And the confessions: I skipped Saturday because I had Oreos.

I kept assuring everyone that I wasn't the food police, that their diet diaries would be anonymous and safe with me. But that didn't matter. One friend suggested that the material I was gathering would be good fodder for a novel, using the diets as the entry point for a women's dieting club, kind of like the Jane Austen Book Club. She thought that one of the characters could be dishonest in her diary, and that could be one plotline. Given the panic the exercise seemed to trigger, I'm sure there was some dishonesty. But I found the reactions to be almost as telling as the diaries themselves. It showed how important food is to women, how personal it is, and how much they have invested in what they eat.

Marie Claire editor Joanna Coles has more than a passing interest in the topic of food and eating and overeating. It's a subject her readers care about. One of the magazine's most popular new columns is called "Big Girl in a Skinny World," written by a five-foot-two, sixteen-stone young woman who chronicles the challenges of loving fashion while being fat. Coles, as the editor, has tried to bring in more food and eating coverage, and she says that one of the subjects that interests her the most is the tipping point, where a woman goes from being a normal weight to being overweight.

I don't know Coles, but we have a funny, small-world connection. A few months ago, a friend in my apartment building asked if I wanted to join her private yoga class one morning, because her regular partner couldn't make it. The class was fantastic, and it turned out that the regular partner was Coles, which I discovered in the course of our interview. We have quite a few other friends in common and had a nice talk in her office in the Hearst Tower. Her office is spacious and sunny, with great views of Manhattan.

Coles tells me that she grew up in England, eating dishes like shepherd's pie, fish and chips, and various roasts and that she's never had a weight issue, although she did recently meet with a nutritionist to figure out how to lose five pounds. As an outsider, she has a good eye for some of the peculiarities of New York eating, and most of her stories revolve around women whose food behaviour ranges from unhappy to unhealthy. In one case, it's a friend who eats little in public but whose car is filled with candy wrappers. She is apparently hiding her calorie intake from her husband, who praises her in public for eating "like a bird." In another, it's a friend who has a mental calorie counter going at all times. At the end of a day, that might mean a spare, 300-calorie supper—not much fun on a dinner date.

At the business functions she attends, Coles says food is treated as a prop rather than as something to be enjoyed or to nourish. Women either make a big deal of ordering a meal and then don't eat it, or they pull what she calls "a *When Harry Met Sally*," fastidiously ordering everything on the side à la Meg Ryan's character in the 1989 film. "It's not like Italy, where real ideas are discussed and you relax into a great feast," says Coles. In general, the Manhattan that Coles inhabits has an uneasy rapport with food.

Although some executives relish an extravagant business lunch at a restaurant like Le Bernardin, the fashion industry lunches to socialize, to make connections, and to be seen in the right restaurants with the right companions. Coles says she is as guilty as the next editor and often just orders whatever her tablemate is having, because studying the menu "seems like a waste of time."

One of her favourite meeting places is Michael's, a midtown media hangout, and I know why. Walk into the dining room at lunchtime and you'll spot half a dozen faces you know from television or from magazine mastheads, if that's your thing. Editor Tina Brown, talk-show host Charlie Rose, media mogul Barry Diller, and fashion legend Anna Wintour are all patrons. So are media investor Michael Fuchs and magazine executive Jack Kliger. You just feel the room's collective antennae perk up when a celebrity sweeps in, looking for a table. (You might also read about such entrances on the restaurant's Twitter feed, where it announces the arrival of its more famous guests).

Dishes from the kitchen, like foie gras and butter-poached lobster, can't really compete with that kind of excitement, and, in fact, the food isn't all that good. Coles says that consulting the menu is an exercise in redundancy. For one thing, people know what they are going to order before they sit down—and it's not the foie gras. "We all know we're having the Cobb salad. Most know they'll have it without the bacon and without the cheese," Coles tells me. What do you expect, she asks. "No one goes to Michael's for food," she says. "You go for the energy in the room."

* *

Training the Brain

Here are some dos and don'ts and principles from veteran New York eaters:

Manhattan Diet Dos

❏ Always leave a little on your plate. It can even be small, a crumb; just be aware you're doing it, and watch it go into the garbage.

❏ Chunky is better than smooth.

❏ Warm is better than cold.

❏ Fat is better than no fat.

❏ Dilute! Use water, soda water, ice.

Manhattan Diet Don'ts

❏ Never eat anything that comes wrapped in plastic.

❏ Don't get too thirsty.

❏ Don't eat anything that is disguised to look better than it is.

❏ Never eat while in motion, not walking or in a car.

❏ Don't get really, really hungry.

❏ Cut out diet fizzy drinks except when you have a sore throat.

❏ Never drink coffee, even decaf, when you're hungry or at night! It always eventually makes you more hungry.

Expert recipes derived from the above principles in no particular order include:

❑ Eat a spoonful or two of peanut butter or almond butter when you're hungry.

❑ Have a cheese stick.

❑ Add milk to green tea. It tastes like melted green-tea ice cream.

❑ Spread avocado thin, like butter, on wholemeal toast.

❑ Drink warm skimmed milk before going to bed.

❑ Drink red wine—that is, if you don't have a problem with alcohol. Unless it's fancy, dilute it with soda water and a drop of pomegranate juice—and even ice.

❑ Eat soup. Melt a little cheese in the soup.

❑ Before having a restaurant meal, eat olives.

❑ Add peanuts, avocado, or cheese to salads.

❑ Microwave an apple.

❑ Microwave or steam all vegetables, and add parmesan and/or olive oil. Eat them warm.

. . . .

So what it is it about the Manhattanite's thought process that keeps her fit? One of the most well-known books on the topic of what prompts people to overeat is the 1974 book *Obese Humans and Rats* by Stanley Schachter and Judith Rodin. In it, the researchers describe how they spent thousands of hours combing through studies and found that some of the factors that make rats fat can make humans fat, too. Their conclusion: the more work it takes to eat something, the less we eat. Given the option of opening a bag of corn chips or the task of husking corn, slicing it off the cob, and roasting it, guess what the over-eater picks?

And it's not just obvious examples like that. Wansink, the Cornell professor mentioned earlier, has measured how much more ice cream diners ate when the lid of a cafeteria cooler was left open rather than shut, and how much more milk they drank when the milk dispenser was closer to the dining area. When Wansink gave secretaries Hershey's Kisses in two ways—either on their desks or about six feet away—those who had the chocolates within reach ate 5.6 more kisses than their colleagues who had to get up.

In my opinion, living in Manhattan is like a full-time Wansink experiment. With seven thousand restaurants here, one for every 220 inhabitants, there is the equivalent of a giant glass candy bowl on every corner. And that number doesn't included delis, ice cream parlours, candy shops, pizza joints, or street carts. In theory, the abundance of food should be a fat sentence for each and every Manhattanite. Yet it's not, partly because people train themselves not to eat, partly because of an excess of choice, and partly because of the influence of fashion, friends, and strangers.

Wansink chalks it up to the extra number of decisions a consumer has to make to actually purchase something. He gives the example of jelly beans. If there is a bowl of them in your home, the only decision is whether to cross the room and take a handful. Do you really want the calories? But when you are walking down the street and come across a jelly bean store, you have to cross both a physical and a metaphysical door. On the physical level is the candy shop entrance. On the metaphysical level, you have to decide if you want the calories *that* much, if you want to shell out three dollars for a bag of candy, and if you have the time to purchase the candy, thereby making you late for wherever you are going. That's four decisions instead of one, he says—a pretty strong deterrent. It's maths that at least partly explains why New Yorkers don't pop into every Starbucks they pass or grab a frankfurter every time they go by a hot dog cart.

New Yorkers choose to describe this behavior as discipline, as putting blinders on, and as training themselves. *Discipline*, in fact, is a word that comes up again and again in interviews: "There's nothing wrong with a little discipline," or "I'm disciplined," or "It's all about discipline." In this version of Manhattan, ice cream, pizza, and candy all become part of the city's background noise to be blocked out. It is part of the constant food editing that occupies a special place in our brains. It's watching every piece of food that goes in your mouth. It is an exhausting mindfulness. Yet it works better than pills. It's been proven scientifically. In one unpublished study I read, mindful eaters lost an average of 10 pounds in a year, more than what was lost in trials of weight-loss drugs. To think like a New York eater, you have to listen to your inner eater. It might be tiring, but it will get you through the rough spots.

Manhattan Diet Secrets

- ❏ *Manhattan women don't eat in the moment.* You shouldn't, either. Come up with a grand scheme that spans meals and days. If you overindulge in the morning, pull back at night. Or if you go crazy over the weekend, go spartan on Monday, Tuesday, and Wednesday. Did you have a big barbecue on Friday night? Cut back during the week.

- ❏ *A good meal is not a big meal.* A good meal is one that tastes good. Let Patricia Duffy be your guide. A salad and half a dozen boiled prawns will just leave you feeling very hungry. Go for foods that are satisfying and gratifying. If that's macaroni cheese, so be it. But eat half a portion.

- ❏ *Stop before you're full—way before.* Learn to recognize the sweet spot between not being full and not being hungry.

- ❏ *Make it easy.* If it's easier to eat potato crisps than baked potatoes, save yourself the effort. Don't buy the crisps. Stock the pantry and fridge with stuff you like but that won't send you binging.

- ❏ *Buy small.* Small bags of pretzels, small containers of yogurt, small everything. It will help with portion control and make you more aware of what you're eating. Your brain will register a difference between ripping open ten mini bags of M&M's and opening just one mega bag.

❏ *Seek out peer pressure.* Manhattan is all about being skinny, but what do you do if you live in a place where fat is where it's at? My guess is that even if your friends are overweight, you can find motivation in a Curves gym or a Zumba fitness class. Communal dressing rooms can be highly effective—at least they are for me. I leave one of two ways: horrified by thinking, "Do I look like her?", or pumped by thinking, "Now, that's what I want to look like!" Either way, it's good.

3

Dark Chocolate, Almonds, and Discipline

How We Eat

It was a rainy Thursday night, and New York's foodie pashas were gathered to pay tribute to Ruth Reichl, the editor of *Gourmet* magazine. Reichl's glossy monthly had abruptly folded a week earlier, and now more than two hundred culinary swells—from writer Calvin Trillin to chocolatier Jacques Torres—were jimmied into a private party room to both celebrate her tenure and mourn the loss of an industry touchstone. I was my husband's "plus one."

Naturally, the hors d'oeuvres were impressive, like the guest list. In one corner, a table was laid with an artful selection of olives brined in orange, spiced edamame, and marinated onions and peppers. I watched waiters circulating with thumb-sized nuggets of crisped pork belly, graced with slivers of fresh fig, and salty Swiss chard dumplings topped with wafers of prosciutto. Some offered trays of delicate fried rice balls or mouth-ready bites of hamachi in spoons. All the partyers had to do was open, chew, and swallow.

The funny thing is, hardly anyone did. True to an unspoken New York cocktail etiquette, few guests indulged in more than three or four tastes. Mr. Torres nibbled on almonds from his pocket. Mr. Trillin sampled a ladle of hamachi. Ms. Reichl seemed to not try anything at all.

"This food is good," Cesare said to me, a little sadly. "But New Yorkers don't eat."

Or do they? Many of Ms. Reichl's friends had after-party dinner plans and were pacing themselves. Some were headed to Cesare's place, a few blocks north. Others were on their way downtown to a new hot spot in Chinatown; still others planned to move on to restaurants—Per Se, Masa, A Voce—inside the Time Warner Center, where the party had been held. As though by a secretly understood code, the guests seemed to have agreed ahead of time on one thing: they weren't going to blow dinner later on a couple of mouthfuls now.

After Manhattan's women have been peer-pressured into being fit and thin, after they've done the mental maths about what they should and shouldn't consume, what is it that goes into their mouths? Are they just superhuman when it comes to discipline? Just one big leafy-greens-and-grains, sushi-eating tribe? I don't believe it.

And this is why: I asked dozens of women to keep food diaries, so I *know* what they eat. It's not just the good-for-you stuff that grocery stores sell in the organics aisle, although there is plenty of that. And it's not all just Weight Watchers, point-perfect meals and four-star slivers of yellowfin carpaccio, although there's that, too. Just like the rest of America, Manhattan women eat the kind of unwhole food products that give followers of food writer Michael Pollan the heebie-jeebies. Manhattan women have been known to eat I Can't Believe It's Not Butter and Skinny Cow ice creams Bars. They treat themselves with lollipops and Frosted

Mini-Wheats. For the most part, they don't seem to believe in deprivation at all. Women eat all day long: multiple snacks, meals, treats. There's a lot of yogurt, a lot of cheese, a *lot* of energy bars, and ice cream; a lot of dark chocolate, a lot of almonds, a lot of hummus, and a lot of Starbucks cappuccino.

Some, of course, are so hell-bent on calorie counting they tote cans of water-packed tuna to business lunches, live on a no-carb diet for years on end, or forsake food for protein shakes and nutrition supplements. But here's the catch: mostly there's balance.

It's as though Manhattan Dieters have an inner clock that maintains an equilibrium on a variety of fronts. The women who go crazy overeating at one meal, on one day, or even for one week instinctively cut back at the next meal, on the next day, or for the next week. They keep their eating on the early side of the day rather than the late to give their bodies time to digest. They have an inner voice that directs them to vegetables over bread, good fats over bad ones, and high-fibre meals over low. Those Frosted Mini-Wheats are a miniature portion—just a handful. Somehow, the Manhattan Dieter manages to eat just one lollipop. And she doesn't forget about it. A handful of liquorice comfits at four in the afternoon means no sweets after dinner.

. . . .

What Do You Eat When No One Is Looking?

Nancy Farkas, corporate lawyer: "Late at night, I will have two peanut butter sandwiches and a glass of wine."

Kim Shapiro, hedge fund administrator: "I ate a whole bag of dried pineapple rings. I decided not to buy them again because they are full of sugar. If I have a weakness, it's these dried fruit things. I could eat them and eat them."

Lauren Lipton, novelist: "Good & Plenty. Not the whole bag."

Lori Schwarz, fashion rep: "I buy a box of cherry Pop-Tarts

and split it with my daughter. We eat the box over three days."

Lillie Rosenthal, osteopath: "A Crystal Lite slurpee (like a Slush Puppy) from 7-Eleven. Any flavour."

Debi Wisch, entrepreneur: "Swedish fish candy, just not forty-five of them."

Theresa Passarelli, commercial property manager: "Marshmallows and Nutella."

. . . .

A word of caution. Don't bring up mindfulness, self-control, or discipline with expert types: epidemiologists, sociologists, or whatever kind of academic you think might have a valid opinion here. If you do, you'll get an earful about what Manhattanites eat to get thin. They'll get all righteous and say there's nothing special about Manhattan that makes the citizens fit. Instead, they'll talk about food choices and the availability of groceries and how the more food choices there are in a place, the skinnier the people are who live there—as though the only reason Manhattanites are thinner than residents in the other four New York boroughs is the 322 supermarkets between Battery Park and 155th Street.

The experts will also chalk up Manhattan fitness to wealth. A Manhattanite, they'll note, can afford to pay a couple of dollars for a single serving of Greek yogurt or for an organic apple with a Barbie-sized carbon footprint. It's like I'm in a different conversation. "Are you listening?" I want to ask. "That's not what I'm talking about." Yes, Manhattan is wealthy. Okay, people in poorer neighbourhoods tend to be more overweight because they have fewer supermarkets. And unfortunately, people there have to shop at 7-Elevens and other convenience stores, where there are no leafy greens, wholegrains, or fish.

Yet in the neighbourhoods I frequent, there is a totally different issue, however frivolous it may seem to you. Here in the land of über-plenty and softball-sized muffins, the challenge is restraint. Here the problem is eating skinny in the fat zone. So what's the secret?

After interviewing more than a hundred women, specialists, doctors, nutritionists, chefs, grocery store cashiers, waiters, and others, I've concluded it comes down to two things: training and cheating. It's that simple. The Manhattanites I'm talking about have conditioned themselves to not want the street food, crisps, and menu distractions like hot fudge sundaes. At the same time, they've figured out the treats that won't derail them totally if they have one in the late afternoon.

This doesn't square with the mindless-eating theories of Cornell's Professor Brian Wansink. He says people are not so mindless when it comes to street food and candy shops because of inhibitors—having to break stride to enter a store, the money-spending issue, and complications like not wanting to be late for an appointment. All of that may very well be true and probably plays a role. But none of the women I interviewed mentioned any of those factors. Instead, they talked about tuning food out, about putting blinders on, about no longer seeing the hot fudge sundae on the menu. These women said they'd just trained themselves. Like Pavlov's dog, but in reverse. By repeatedly not eating things they believe are fattening, too sugary or greasy, or whatever offence fits the bill, they have redirected their taste buds.

The novelist Lauren Lipton was the first to bring it up. I know Lauren from our days at the *Wall Street Journal*, where we sat in adjoining cubicles and both worked on the *Journal*'s weekend life-style section. At that point, Lauren was covering the frothy fashion-and-shopping beat, and I was her editor—a job that mostly involved ginning up statistics and sales figures to bolster her argument that the trend she'd spotted was actually a trend. There were always leggy models with cascading hair around Lauren's desk, zipping up thigh-high boots, slipping on cashmere robes, or tottering around in satiny bedroom mules.

Lauren and I turned out to be kindred souls; we were among the few employees at the *Journal* who knew the difference between Gianni Versace and Giorgio Armani. We could discuss clothes endlessly. But it wasn't until I started working on this book that I realized Lauren was a diet obsessive, too. She has a ballerina's body, all long limbs, and a milky complexion. I always assumed she was just blessed with good genes and a fast metabolism. Both are true, she says. But she also works at it.

Lauren's training started early, when her mom, a hippie in 1970s California, told her that if she chose an apple instead of a chocolate chip cookie for dessert, she wouldn't have pimples as a teenager. Lauren took the lesson to heart and began drilling cookie cravings out of her system. It's been years since she salivated at the sight of a cookie jar, a bag of crisps, a Milky Way bar, or a pouf of candy floss. And the work has been so thorough, so expert, that she doesn't think of not eating those things as depriving herself. She fills up on really healthy stuff: fruit early in the morning and porridge for breakfast; a burrito or a salad for lunch; beans and wholewheat pasta with kale and spring greens sautéed in olive oil and garlic for dinner.

So virtuous! So nutritious! So boring, you might say! Ah, but there's cheating, too. And this is the key, because it's what keeps a lot of women I talked to sane. They eat portion-controlled amounts of high-sugar, low-fat, junky candy. In Lauren's case it's liquorice comfits, which she keeps in small bags in her kitchen.

. . . .

How They Diet

ANNA WINTOUR

Vogue's legendary editor-in-chief, Anna Wintour, maintains her model-thinness through a power lunch consisting of rare red meat and a salad with no salad dressing.

. . . .

I heard a lot about this sort of thing from other women. They like lollipops, liquorice, Gobstoppers, Mary Janes peanut butter chews, and Gummy Bears—gummy anything. I'm not talking about saturated-fat offenders like Butterfingers or Twix bars. I'm not talking about expensive dark chocolate, although that has its fans. I mean cheap sugary candy! It goes back to the food bravado I talked about in chapter 2. Candy seems decadent. But at about 100 calories for 25 grams, it really isn't so bad. It's more like an enabler. It allows women to stay on message, dietwise: trained yet sweet-tooth satisfied.

I consider the actress Christine Baranski to be self-trained. I met Christine at my friend Dorothy Hamilton's weekend house a few summers ago. We had a long languorous lunch on Dorothy's dock, overlooking Lake Waramug in Connecticut, with a few others, including Maria Campbell, a literary agent who secures book rights for Warner Bros. Pictures. It was a perfect afternoon. It would have been Gatsbyesque, if we had been on Long Island instead of in northwest Connecticut. Dorothy, as she always does, served spectacularly sumptuous food: a gorgeous gazpacho bursting with tomatoes, peppers, and garlic from her garden; an obscenely lavish salad with Sardinian tuna and Niçoise olives; and hunks of freshly baked French bread. If you'd snapped a photo of the table, it could have been a four-colour brochure for a local bed-and-breakfast. Christine really ate; she didn't just push food around on her plate. Still, I pegged her as a Manhattan Dieter, and it turns out I was right.

Theatre, movie, and television buffs will know that Christine has pretty much been thin—five feet eight, nine and a half stone— her whole career. Except for a one-and-a-half-stone blip the first few months she was enrolled at Juilliard, she says she never had a pudgy period or an up-and-down thing. Staying slim is just what she's always done.

It could have been different. Back in Buffalo, where she grew up, Christine was weaned on hearty, home-cooked Polish food— her mom's sausage and pierogi and homemade doughnuts. But for an aspiring actress, being fat wasn't an option, so instead she put food on the back burner. She never was interested in cooking—or eating, for that matter—although she likes making curried squash bisque and pumpkin bread for friends and spending days in the kitchen with her daughters getting ready for Christmas. Typically, Christine says, she eats only two meals a day, with a late snack in lieu of lunch. Breakfast is a protein shake with blueberries, almond milk, and Spirateen, a soya-based protein powder. Sometimes when she's working in a play, she forgets to stop for a meal altogether. "I'm moderate," says the fifty-eight-year-old.

For example, after leaving a concert at Carnegie Hall recently, she popped into Petrossian, a Russian restaurant known for its caviar, and had a cup of borscht, a bit of smoked salmon, and a glass of wine. "My eating is more like a French woman's," she says. "If I do indulge or if I'm in a situation where I go out a lot, the next week I'll pull back."

Christine and I are swapping diet stories at Via Quadronno, an Italian coffee and sandwich shop on the Upper East Side near her apartment. Via Quadronno is one of the area's de facto salons, serving a decent cappuccino in a room that's done up in vaguely Tyrolean accents. Stop by the restaurant at any time of day, and you'll note society ladies parked on the velveteen banquettes in the back, sipping espresso and Splenda and not eating their rocket salads. In her simple black trousers and sweater, Christine fits right in, looking much as she does in *The Good Wife*, in which she plays a power litigator who commands the office in slinky wrap dresses and expensive suits. Christine actually thinks that one reason her career has lasted so long is that clothes fit her well.

Late at night, Christine's idea of the perfect snack is a bowl of granola with milk. When she goes out to dinner with her husband, she orders grilled salmon with spinach and rice. At Swifty's, an Upper East Side society haunt, it's calf liver. At a splurge dinner at Del Posto, an Italian restaurant that recently won a four-star review, she had a small plate of pumpkin ravioli and a green salad. "That sufficed," she says. "If I'm working late, I will allow myself a treat,"—there it is again—"a little piece of chocolate cake. But I don't finish it. I just take a few bites. I said I didn't watch my weight, but I guess I do." Her standby vice is dark chocolate, which she says she is very happy to have discovered.

So—training and cheating. It's very yin–yang. But it also rings true. Christine tells me she's got friends who say they lose the taste for white sugar and refined flour after not eating it for a while, and she knows the feeling. In behaviour modification theory, it takes twenty-eight days to change a behaviour, or so I've read. If you can go twenty-eight days without a can of Easy Cheese, the next twenty-eight days without Easy Cheese will be easier. And so on. Of course, if it were that easy, there would be no need for diets and diet books. It goes against human nature not to eat something you like.

But I try to think about it this way: I'm fifty-plus years old. Ten days doesn't add up to much as a percentage of my life. If I can get to day eleven not eating a particular food, I can break the psychological addiction. I think, "What can I do not to have chocolate-covered raisins again?" If I can get through ten days without chocolate-covered raisins, I've passed the detox test. It's like not drinking alcohol for ten days when you're on antibiotics. You don't drink, and it's no big deal, and after ten days you're not thinking about the glass of wine with dinner so much.

As I consider retraining myself, my mind wanders to my dinners with Ruth, Shari, and Dana three or four times a year. These women are good friends, and we get together when we can for a little female bonding. Our meals could be a scene in a "chick flick" starring Catherine Keener or Frances McDormand. We don't talk about dieting as a group, though. It would be too, well, like a "chick flick." Instead, we helicopter around the issue, discussing everything but.

Remember food bravado? Well, when the four of us get together, it's in full flower. The last time this happened we were at a noisy Upper West Side bistro called Five Napkin Burger. The place has a menu that reads like a greatest restaurant hits of the past three decades. There's spinach and artichoke dip, very seventies; chicken wings, very eighties; and sushi, very nineties. Other dishes range from onion rings to burgers to chicken tenders to a foot-long Kobe beef hot dog.

Organizing the outing took nearly a gigabyte of BlackBerry exchanges, mostly because Ruth and Dana are hot-shot executives with their own handlers and are hard to pin down.

We arrived one by one, with a flurry of kisses, stories, and news. The normal things were discussed: family, work, current events, movies, and books. Eating, not at all. But the obsessive in me was taking notes. I scrutinized what we ordered, what we didn't order, and what we actually ate—which in this case was three completely different things. We kicked things off with a bottle of wine. Okay by me. Then someone—no names here—asked the waiter to start the table with the onion rings. This was classic, I thought. Ordering onion rings signals: we're not sissies, we're not girly, we're *eaters*. On cue, we all oohed. We all aahed. And when the dish arrived, we each grabbed one onion ring—and nibbled. The rest of the onion rings stayed on the plate, uneaten.

There was also an order of the spinach and artichoke dip. No takers there, either. And an untouched bread basket.

Ruth, Shari, and Dana all chose ahi tuna burgers, which came on a bed of mixed leaves and seems to live on the menu for women like us. I went with sushi, what I refer to as the default dinner. For dessert, we split a cheesecake about the size of a beer coaster—one healthy forkful or so apiece.

Going home, I thought, so this is how Manhattan eats. It wouldn't be dinner without a bottle of wine, and among four of us, that's one generous glass each. There are the onion rings and spinach dip for show. That's okay. No one touched the bread. What we actually ate was fish and salad—and a forkful of dessert. Ha! We are so trained, it's scary.

Of course, how I eat in a restaurant with friends isn't necessarily how I eat on my own, especially when I'm alone in my apartment, out running errands, or heading for work. At the time of our dinner, I was on a cinnamon doughnut kick. Three or so times a week, before I got to my office in the morning, I'd stop at a doughnut cart and get a cinnamon doughnut the size of an aubergine and a large coffee, and that would be my breakfast and lunch. One day I woke up and thought, "This is insane! And unhealthy!" I'd gained five pounds. So I stopped. Twenty-eight days came and went with no cinnamon doughnut. And I haven't had one since. It worked! Trained again!

In 2008, when Mayor Michael Bloomberg decided to shock and awe his subjects with calorie postings in fast-food restaurants, two things happened. In the city's lower-income neighbourhoods, people started ordering more calories. That was unexpected. Apparently, they started using the new calorie counts to help them choose the food with the most bang for the buck.

But the Manhattan Dieters in the four-dollar-a-cup (£2.50) coffee world had a different reaction. They freaked out. A Starbucks Hazelnut Signature Hot Chocolate with whipped cream has 860 calories? An apple fritter is 490 calories? Once that information was on display, the average number of calories per order at Starbucks fell like a deflated latte—by 14 percent! Manhattanites with a little extra cash not only started buying fewer items, they also started ordering less fattening stuff.

Bad for business, you might think. But at Starbucks shops located within about three hundred feet of Dunkin' Donuts shops, revenues actually went up. My explanation: once waist watchers realized how many calories were in a doughnut, they decided to move their consumption to a place with a little more social cachet.

Should I be embarrassed to say it? These are my people—the slice of Manhattan that downgrades calories and upgrades location. Manhattan attracts upwardly mobile, ambitious people, and they are just as zealous in their diet lives as in their professional ones. I asked Dr. Anna Fels, a New York psychiatrist who studies ambition in women, about this. Latte lovers (my stand-in for an upper socioeconomic demographic) tend to be more disciplined in most areas of their lives, says Dr. Fels. "Delayed gratification is a bigger part of how they live. They are drawn to diet and exercise and healthy choices because the discipline can give the women a sense of control."

"Look," she explains, "women who are successful profession-ally are shrewd enough to know that appearance matters. Ergo, they work at it. If you look at women CEOs, you rarely see the Lloyd Blankfein equivalent in a woman CEO," she says, referring to the lumpy-looking head of Goldman Sachs. "Men's looks count, but not in the same way [as] for women."

I have a highly accomplished friend who is totally on board with this theory. Being thin in career-oriented Manhattan is an asset, she says, as it is in most places. "You get recruited [for a job], so life is the message. If you're fat, it's not going to help you." And it goes beyond that. My pal sees being thin here as a sign of character strength. It tells the world you have self-control and discipline.

"There's a sense of superiority," she says. My friend doesn't want her name mentioned for a variety of reasons. My friend is beautiful. She's got perfect posture and a killer bod. She could wear a Walmart suit and you'd think it was Dolce & Gabbana. I don't know how she does it. Well, I do. She runs six to seven miles a day, and her food obsession is deeper and broader and more ingrained than mine.

Her neuroses don't really show their true colours when she eats in public with friends. There, she merely seems careful: salad without dressing, spinach without oil, that sort of thing. But it's like me and my cinnamon doughnuts. When left to her own devices, this highly accomplished friend of mine eats differently—except she doesn't eat cinnamon doughnuts. In fact, if there were cinnamon doughnuts in her apartment, she'd throw them in the garbage, then pour water on them just to make sure she didn't try one.

This is the woman who used to bring water-packed tuna in a can to business meetings. When she left New York for a year and couldn't find fat-free Greek yogurt in local supermarkets, she had it shipped. In spite of her running regimen, she keeps her daily intake to between 1,200 and 1,300 calories. She doesn't keep anything vaguely tempting in her home kitchen, including energy bars and breakfast cereal. If her fiancé brings cookies or other treats home, she throws them away after he leaves or—I wasn't joking—pours water on them. "I have a mental counter on all the time," she says. "It's not normal. I wouldn't recommend it."

So what does this highly accomplished woman eat? Not much. She starts her day with low-fat yogurt and almonds or an egg-white omelette. She has an apple or an orange as a mid-morning snack, then a salad for lunch, without dressing or anything on it that's remotely fattening. She'll have another piece of fruit in the afternoon and a can of tuna on salad for dinner, with some mandarin oranges as dessert. It's pretty much always been that way, even when she was a teenager. (Caveat: she does let down her guard sometimes, because I've seen her eating focaccia and chunks of Parmigiano-Reggiano at parties.)

About ten years ago, when my friend was feeling a little lethargic, she met with a nutritionist who encouraged her to write down the calories of what she ate and how much she exercised each day. And she did. For three years! (When I asked my volunteers to write down what they ate for a week, I got some grumbles.) She has hundreds of spreadsheets in a notebook, and she showed them to me. She doesn't keep the count any more, unless she feels the need. But she still brings her own food when she visits friends for the weekend. She knows it's over the top, but it's also just her.

"I don't cheat," she says. "If you want to make it happen, you make it happen."

. . . .

New York Stories

Nathalie Kirsheh, Art Director

Natalie has lost more thabn three stone over the last year and a half, and she's still working at it. She likes the challenge of dieting and has completely given up cheese, which was hard because her family is Mediterranean and dairy was always a big part of her diet. She likes for the waiter in a restaurant to bring a bread basket, so she can see how long she can resist. "It's an achievement," she says. "By stopping after one piece, it's like you're able to control it."

Robin Reif, Marketing Executive

Robin is like a calculator. She knows the calories of everything that goes into her mouth, from the egg salad half sandwich she orders from Pret a Manger every day (285) to the peanut crunch diet bars she snacks on (180). When she approaches a fast-food outlet, the thought of entering never crosses her mind. "It's out of the question," she says. "I would never go into Dunkin' Donuts unless I was desperate for coffee. I wouldn't go into Baskin Rob-bins. I never get anything at Starbucks except for coffee."

. . . .

Not even my very accomplished friend would suggest that other people should eat as she does, but her example proves that how you eat is not just a question of money and supermarket access. Diet dis-cipline is a state of mind, and there are a lot of Manhattanites who share it. This is not just a New York City phenomenon. There is a group consciousness shared by thin women everywhere. You're either in the bubble or out of it. In the bubble, the care and feeding of a slim figure becomes a sixth sense. You are as alert to diet busters as to mug-gers or wayward cars. Out of the bubble, a third fudge brownie is no different from the second one. It's a sense of proportion and vigilance that you carry with you all the time.

The problem is when discipline leaves joy behind. A lot of dieters have that issue. It's just sad. Food is not the enemy. It's not even the frenemy. But you might not know that from poking around in refrigerators and grocery stores. Witness the catalogue of non-foods in Manhattan that cater to the eating neurotics. I understand the lite beer and the Frosted Mini-Wheats. I even get turkey bacon and other food facsimiles. But what has no place in the Manhattan Diet is the plastic—a product meant to resemble some actual food but in which the taste has been zapped out.

For instance, those baby carrots that you see everywhere. There's nothing "baby" about them. They're inch-long stubs, cut out of abnormally large carrots, in the guise of convenience. And then they're packed into 500-gram bags that you find in practically every grocery store and deli, with 175 calories, 0 grams of fat or cholesterol, and 0 grams of flavour per bag. I guess because the upside is they're already peeled. But did you ever buy them? They're so far from carrots they could be watermelon rind, just not as tasty. They're old, discoloured, and waterlogged.

Same for the take-out sushi available at checkout counters all over the city. Fresh sushi is a no-brainer diet food. But sushi in a plastic box in an open refrigerator case near the cash register is an invitation to bacterial disaster.

And then there's Tasti D-Lite. You probably have a variation of this where you live. Tasti D-Lite is a frozen dessert sold out of tiny storefronts around the city and made from, among other things, skimmed milk, sugar, corn syrup, cream, guar gum, locust bean gum, and carrageenan. There are practically more ingredients than calories, which total fewer than 25 an ounce, depending on the flavour. Back in 2004, Tasti D-Lite had a fleeting moment of national fame when it was featured in an episode of *Sex and the City*. Today it lives on, fuelling the practice of nutritionists whose clients consider it a meal substitute. If you're going to eat a processed food, at least pick something that satisfies a craving or hits a sweet spot. It's too depressing to waste calories on bad diet food.

Yet truth be told, in doing my research I met a lot of women who ate this stuff and worse, embracing food about as joyfully as a pat-down at the airport. I especially saw it in the fashion crowd, where magazine editors, models, and bookers pad their low-cal habits with diet supplements and energy drinks. They eat a lot of egg-white omelettes, plain pitta, and plain yogurt and consider food a foe. A few years back, I remember, *New York* magazine asked Anne Slowey, an editor of *Elle*, to track her diet for three days during Fashion Week.

On day one, the "food" Slowey ate consisted of a serving of eggs and an iced skinny latte in the morning, a glass of wine at two in the afternoon, and two glasses of red wine, Camembert cheese on crackers, and three olives for dinner. The rest of her nutrition was delivered through energy drinks and other supplements. Day two was almost identical, with Slowey subsisting on a bowl of vegetable soup, an organic food bar, a tiny portion of ceviche, guacamole and chips, a few glasses of champagne, and a beer. The reaction in the blogosphere was swift and harsh: Slowey's diet was "anorexic." Not that it mattered. Slowey is still at *Elle*, even more famous than ever, thanks to a stint on the television show *Stylista*.

I didn't talk to Slowey, but she seems the extreme, far from the training-and-cheating paradigm. But her habits do point to the other unsaid operating factor: money. The poor, as my epidemiology pals will quickly point out, don't typically try to squeak by on a couple of mouthfuls of ceviche, guacamole, and another assorted 500 calories a day. Manhattan is a money town, and anyone buying organic, dabbling in juice fasts, or eating any of the foods I've mentioned in this chapter is pretty much rolling in it. Dieting Manhattan style is a well-off person's indulgence. Whole Foods didn't earn the nickname Whole Paycheck for nothing. Christine's orange juice at Via Quadronno was $5 (£3), and my smallish cappuccino was $4.50 (£2.80)—pricier even than Starbucks. The tuna that the banker uses to dress her salad is a dollar an ounce and is shipped to her from California.

The money angle runs through my mind as I am talking to Debi Wisch, the friend of a friend who lives on Fifth Avenue in an apartment I can only describe as palatial. There are sweeping views of Central Park, and the art is all name brand. Everything is airy, light-filled, tasteful, and perfect—just like Debi. She is one of the fittest forty-six-year olds I've ever met, five feet four and just under eight stone. She says that she has the arms of a twenty-something, and to prove it, she drops to the floor during our talk and starts doing push-ups and other exercises, including a yoga position called *vasisthasana* that I've tried for twelve years to master but still don't have the upper body strength to pull off. (If you're curious: the move involves propping yourself up sideways like a plank, with your heels pressing the floor, your legs straight and stiff, and most of your weight resting on one arm.)

Debi runs a one-of-a-kind jewellery business with designer Janis Provisor, and before that she had her own fashion public relations firm. She's not much of a foodie, but she clearly has the means to eat well and does. Her husband is a cancer survivor, and since his recovery a few years ago, Debi tells me, she's redoubled her efforts to eat organic, whole, and unprocessed foods.

You should see her kitchen. It could be its own wing of Whole Foods. She snaps open drawer after drawer, and within each is a distinct trove of organically correct snacks. The first is filled with nuts and dried fruit. There are cashews dusted with curry and cashews sprinkled with sugar. There are bags of almonds, pistachios, raisins in half a dozen shades and shapes, dried cranberries, and dried edamame with wasabi. A second drawer is stocked with energy bars, some from Quaker Oats, some high-fibre varieties from Gnu, Clif Bars, high-fibre crackers, and other crunchy, salty snacks. There are also bags of dark chocolate—no M&M's or Snickers bars. None of the stash is necessarily low-fat, but there's nary a calorie that wouldn't pass muster with the food police.

"I try not to be crazy," Debi says. "I have two daughters, and I don't want them having eating disorders. I want them to eat everything."

It would be lovely if everyone could afford to eat this way. No one ever said the Manhattan Diet would be cheap. In a perfect world, Debi's diet would be the Manhattan Diet. It's sane, balanced, and healthy. If her kids are going to eat something sweet, she tells them it should be something they really enjoy. If that happens to be a cupcake, it should be a fantastic cupcake from Magnolia Bakery.

For herself, Debi loosely follows the F-Factor regimen, a diet by New York's nutritionist of the moment, Tanya Zuckerbrot, who emphasizes high fibre, high protein, and lots of wholegrain crispbread, "the appetite-control cracker." For breakfast that means Greek yogurt with berries and fibre cereal. Lunch is a salad or a wrap. Dinner is fish and vegetables. She snacks a lot, on cashews or blueberries, not junk food; if she wants something sweet, she grabs a small piece of candy.

There's nothing to criticize. It's perfect. When she entertains, she puts out lollipops for her guests. She doesn't like pasta, but if she wants a carb fix, she'll have a muffin. She's not crazy for chocolate, but she loves liquorice and keeps a stock of it at home. She doesn't believe in denying herself. "I'm appalled when forty-five-year old women sit around at lunch and discuss what not to eat," she says. "I try 90 percent of the time to be good and the other 10 percent just to enjoy."

I am hoping that Debi puts me on the invitation list for her next dinner party. The menu for a recent one included chicken tagine, roasted salmon, and wheat-berry salad, among other dishes. But the showstopper was dessert, which starred sweets from all of Debi's favourite bakeries around the city. There was a velvet cake from Cakeman Raven, a bakery in Brooklyn; a peanut butter pie from Billy's, a sweet shop in Chelsea; a Magnolia Bakery coconut cake; and a chocolate confection from the confidently named Best

Chocolate Cake in the World shop in SoHo. She tells me that her friends were amazed. I'm sure they were. She wins hands down on the food bravado front. Brava, Debi.

As part of my research into how Manhattan women eat, I asked twenty-five slim, fit women with a healthy attitude towards eating (no crazy food issues or food fears) to keep a food diary for a week. For the most part, the women were between thirty-five and sixty-five, with two women in their twenties. I asked my volunteers to write down everything they ate and the time and any exercise they might have done during the day. Here is a peek inside five very different entries.

Diary 1: Forty-Two-Year-Old Journalist

1-mile walk to school. At least 2 more to and from office and errands. Gym: 75 minutes (about 7.5 miles) on the elliptical trainer, then about 10 to 15 minutes doing stretches and stomach exercises.

8:45 a.m.
1 cup coffee with whole milk

11:00 a.m.
1 hard candy

12:30 p.m.
1 Pret a Manger roast beef baguette (580 calories: roast beef, mayo, mustard, rocket, parmesan)
10 red grapes
1 can Fresca (fizzy grapefruit drink)

5:00 p.m.
1 large pear
1 1-inch cube Swiss cheese
¼ litre water

6:15 p.m.
1 bar of chocolate chip cookie dough (220 calories; ingredients: cashews, dates, chocolate chips, salt)

8:30 p.m.
> 225g leftover bean, soya sausage, and rice concoc-
> tion from last night, topped with 1 tablespoon grated
> reduced-fat Monterey Jack cheese
>
> 225g cooked sliced greens sautéed with 2 tablespoons
> olive oil, 1 clove garlic, 1 tablespoon red wine vinegar,
> ⅛ teaspoon salt
>
> 1 slice wholemeal toast with 2 teaspoons butter
>
> Handful of M&M's
>
> ¼ litre water

Diary 2: Thirty-Seven-Year-Old Yoga Teacher

8:30 a.m.
> ½ litre water

8:45 a.m.
> Walked about a mile to Exhale

9:15–10:30 a.m.
> Taught music yoga flow

10:45 a.m.
> ½ litre carrot, grapefruit, and orange juice in a
> smoothie

11:00 a.m.–12:15 p.m.
> Taught level ½ yoga

12:45 p.m.
> Walked to Candle Café
>
> ½ bowl butternut squash
>
> ½ serving breakfast burrito
>
> 175g sautéed broccoli
>
> Walked home, about ½ a mile

3:00 p.m.
> 1 soya milk ice lolly
>
> 3 Reese's Peanut Butter Cups (small ones)

3:30–4:15 p.m.
> Hula rehearsal

5:00–7:05 p.m.
> Taught two yoga classes

8:30 p.m.
> Dinner from Saigon Grill
>> 300g pad thai
>> 1 bowl coconut vermicelli noodle soup
> Dessert from Le Pain Quotidien
>> ½ brownie
>> 1 small slice lemon tart

Diary 3: Sixty-Two-Year-Old Public Relations Professional

8:00 a.m.
> Walked for 1 hour

9:30–10:30 a.m.
> Barre Burn (Pilates, balance class)

10:30–11:30 a.m.
> Move 'n Groove dance class

12:15 p.m.
>> 2 dried peach halves
>> 4 walnuts
>> 10 hazelnuts
>> 1 tablespoon dried cherries
>> large coffee (grande Starbucks—black)

4:00 p.m.
>> 50g chicken
>> 4 cherry tomatoes
>> 100g red leaf lettuce; 1 tablespoon olive oil; sea salt and pepper

6:15 p.m.
   1 carrot

6:20 p.m.
   90ml white wine

6:45 p.m.
   1 carrot, 4 radishes

7:00 p.m.
   90ml red wine

7:22 p.m.
   40g raw fennel; 60g courgette sautéed in oil with basil

7:50 p.m.
   1 2-inch Yukon Gold potato, roasted
   75g carrots, parsnips, and onions, roasted
   2 tablespoons barley

8:15 p.m.
   1 chicken leg—75g without bone
   75g barley
   50g roasted vegetables

9:00 p.m.
   125ml red wine
   1 square dark chocolate

Diary 4: Forty-Two-Year-Old Nurse

7:00 a.m.
   1 cup coffee with 1 tablespoon unsweetened soya milk

7:30 a.m.
   200g brown rice with minced beef and green peas
   1 banana
   ¼ litre water

2:00 p.m.
   Spinach salad with store-bought yogurt dressing

125g hummus with 1 wholemeal pitta
1 litre water

8:00 p.m.
400g artichoke pasta with oil, garlic, and parmesan cheese
¼ litre water with splash of orange juice

9:30 p.m.
3 chocolate chip cookies
250ml unsweetened soya milk

Diary 5: Fifty-One-Year-Old Graphic Designer

9:00 a.m.
1 café latte
1 buttermilk roll

Noon
1 large dinner plate of 1 medium celeriac steamed with
spring greens
25g blackcurrants over white basmati rice with
2 tablespoons extra-virgin olive oil, salt, and pepper
½ litre water

2:30 p.m.
Peeled, sliced apples with peanut butter

5:30 p.m.
Earl Grey Tea
2 chocolate chip cookies

8:30 p.m.
150g baked striped bass
150g steamed celeriac and spring greens
25g blackcurrants
150g steamed white radish with garlic and thyme
1 tablespoon extra-virgin olive oil on veggies
¼ litre water

Manhattan Diet Secrets

- *Get in mental shape.* Baseball players have spring training. Runners train for the marathon. Boxers train for big matches. Yet when it comes to dieting, people think it's simple, that you just start. But you don't. It takes brain power, not just willpower. You can, however, train yourself not to want certain foods. I was a vegetarian for a couple of years as a teenager. I'm not any more, but I rarely eat meat. I just lost the taste for it. If you train yourself, you can re-engineer your taste buds.

- *Start by thinking about your trigger foods.* What do you eat that prompts other bad eating? When you've isolated one thing, try a ten-day detox. Make a commitment not to eat it for ten days. If you can go without it for ten days, you can go another ten. And then another. And then you're going to forget about that food. You'll have broken the cycle. You might eat the food again, but the craving will be gone.

- *Cheat.* Please! This advice might seem counterproductive after a summons to "man up" and get your diet face on, but it's not. A little cheat—a lollipop, a mini Milky Way, a wedge of Brie, whatever your weakness is—can go a long way. It is a psychological reward, like a mini shopping splurge to quell a binge. Just remember lesson one, and train yourself to stop after a bite or two.

- *Don't cut corners.* Trying to stick to 1,000 calories a day or going without carbohydrates is a recipe for failure. You will feel deprived. Manhattan dieting is forever, not just a few days, weeks, or months. Eat with a lifetime in mind, not just a short-term weight goal. This is part of the mental training concept. Imagine yourself a year from now and see if you can imagine yourself still eating the same way. If the answer is yes, you're on the right track.

- *Find your friends.* By friends I mean foods you love that will get you through. I love sushi. I could eat it every night if it weren't so expensive. Find the healthy, satisfying foods that make you feel good thinking about them.

- *Use some elbow grease.* This is the hard part. Eating well takes work, even cooking. But once you learn how to boil brown rice or sauté broccoli with garlic and olive oil, it won't seem so daunting or time-consuming. And you can make big pots so the food lasts. Then create variations and stretch it out. Lentils can become a salad, a soup, or a side dish.

4

Grocery Love
How We Shop

Let us now ride into the belly of the beast.

I am with the lovely actress Jessica Hecht, conscientious Manhattan Dieter, vegetarian, and mother of two. You might recognize Hecht for her work on Broadway (she was nominated for a Tony Award for her role in *A View from the Bridge*) or her appearances on shows like AMC's *Breaking Bad*. But Hecht is probably best known as the lesbian partner of Ross's ex-wife, Carol, on the NBC sitcom *Friends*. At forty-five, Hecht looks much as she did when that show was a pop-culture phenomenon: tall and lean, with flawless skin. She radiates good health, and I'm about to see why. It's in her grocery basket.

Jess and I were introduced by a mutual friend and have started our shopping date at Bouchon Bakery, chef Thomas Keller's jewel box of a snack and breakfast bar in the Time Warner Center. Bouchon is a favourite spot for Upper West Side foodies; it's like a four-star Starbucks with baguettes and éclairs. As we talk, I am surprised at how much the two of us have in common. We're both Americans married to Italians, and both of us have lived in Italy. We are about the same age (I'm seven years older), both Jewish, both mothers of nine-year-olds. We are both interested in food. Her brother lives in China, and my daughter was born in China. My mom was an actress, too.

Now that we've bonded, we're moving to the next phase of our relationship—where I shadow her as she shops for her family of four.

We catch the escalator and move towards our destination: the fifty-nine-thousand-square-foot Whole Foods in the lower level of the Time Warner building near Central Park. Our descent into the gourmet megaplex is a metaphor for transformation. We two harried consumers are whisked from street level, where rushing pedestrians elbow one another out of the way, sirens wail, taxis honk, and the exhaust from city buses fills the air.

Effortlessly, we are deposited in the magic kingdom of Whole Foods, where we are greeted by a display of fresh-cut flowers: orchids, hydrangeas, sunflowers, and roses, all in full bloom. The lighting is soft, and singer Corrine Bailey Rae purrs to us over the speaker system. This is a parallel underworld, composed of good will, organic bounty, handsome farmers, and nine-dollar (around a fiver) fair-trade chocolate. There is a sushi bar, a pizza bar, a cheese corner, and hot and cold prepared foods. The meat counter is wrapped in what looks like a stock-ticker banner, declaring that its contents contain no added hormones and that the animals ate a 100 percent vegetarian diet.

It is here that the Manhattan Diet begins, because to know what Manhattanites eat, all you really need to do is cruise the aisles of the supermarkets and food stores that serve them. Actually, let me back up. The Manhattan Diet really starts with the choice of where to shop. We have more artisanal, ethnic, hand-harvested, oak-roasted, truffle-dusted, free-range, organic, locally grown, and just plain food per capita than any place on the planet. We have boutiques that specialize in products from the Caribbean, East Asia, and even Australia.

There are 322 supermarkets here, one for every 4,800 residents, plus 23 outdoor farmers' markets. The 10011 postcode alone, in Greenwich Village, has a grocery store for every 2,333 residents. There are some well-heeled communities around the country that have just one store for every 14,000 residents; in poorer neighbourhoods, the ratio can be just one store for every 27,000 residents. The grocery-store bounty doesn't just confer bragging rights; it actually makes Manhattanites skinnier. According to research, living closer to a supermarket can result in a lower body mass index because of the healthier food options the store offers.

But for all the advantages the grocery excess confers, it also raises some existential issues: Where do I begin? Am I a foodie or not? Do I want to be a locavore? In the rest of the world, you may be what you eat. In Manhattan, you are where you shop. Jess, for example, chooses Whole Foods because the store carries organic products, the merchandise is generally good, and it's a four-minute walk from her apartment.

So even before Jess has started loading her trolley, she's staked out some philosophical ground. She is committed to good ingredients. She wants her food as unprocessed as possible, and she is opposed to big agribusiness and in favour of local farmers. Shoppers everywhere take similar positions with the simple decision of where to buy milk, and whether to pick up skimmed, semi-skimmed, or whole, and organic or not. In the most generic sense, it is a choice between old-fashioned grocery stores, where you stock up on breakfast cereal, cleaning products, and lettuce, and the market-come-lately that produces mozzarella in situ and carries wholegrain cereals and phosphate-free cleanser.

How They Diet

MARISKA HARGITAY

No chocolate. No Pringles. After the birth of her son, she cut back on dairy, sugar, and wheat. She ate a lot of organic fruits and vegetables and never left home without a bottle of water. She didn't obsess and didn't weigh herself at home, and she took off nearly three stones in three months.

Pragmatists rely on the former—workhorse chains like Food Emporium, which are in almost every neighbourhood and offer convenience. The women I interviewed in Manhattan, on the other hand, tend to patronize the Whole Foods genre of markets with sushi bars, cheese stations, and product concierges. Price warriors, willing to fight for their beluga lentils, head to Fairway. Loyalists of Eli Zabar, one of the deans of the Manhattan food scene, stick to Eli's, the Vinegar Factory, or E.A.T. The customers of Dean & DeLuca are downtown types who've been overpaying for baby vegetables and housewares in SoHo since before the dawn of Pottery Barn.

As I mentioned, Jess comes to the Time Warner Whole Foods mostly because it's close to her apartment. She shops solo and has to be able to carry whatever she buys. But proximity is not the only factor. Jess could just as easily go two blocks south, to the more mundane Morton Williams Supermarket on West 57th Street. That store, though, doesn't cater to shoppers like her.

Whole Foods is laid out well and has flattering lighting. It helps busy customers by offering half a dozen boxes of pre-chopped vegetable mixes to serve as a base for different soups. It sells healthy-sounding ready-to-heat meals. It stocks conventional and organic versions of most products. There is unsweetened organic soya milk, finely ground organic flaxseed, and vegan gummy candy. Jess likes the recipes Whole Foods puts on its store brands and the fact that she can get almost everything in one store without having to run around to multiple markets.

Yet, oh, the compromises! As we roll past the red potatoes, I merely think, "Red potatoes." But Jess sees them as a potential red flag. They could be from someplace far off, like California. Or worse, Chile. The problem, she explains, is that the market is so well stocked, it's hard to know where items come from. In Italy, where she taught an acting class last year, you know where you are by what's in the fruit and vegetable stand. Tomatoes? The south. Green beans? The north. Whole Foods is more like Esperanto. Those red potatoes could have been flown in from half a dozen different countries—a possibility that doesn't square with her locavore convictions.

Organic products bring up similar dilemmas. Yes, they're healthier and better for the environment. But Jess can't always stomach the high prices, and sometimes the products look worse for the wear. We pause in the fruit section. Jess tells me she likes including a banana in her fourth-grade son's lunch box. If it's got so much as a blemish on it, though, he won't touch it. After examining the conventional and organic choices, she settles on the prettier, non-organic bunch.

And so it goes, with one principle battling another at every stop along the way. Jess would like to mince her own vegetables to make a soup base, but her kitchen is so tiny, it is just easier to use Whole Foods's $5 (£3) box of prechopped celery, carrots, and onions. She doesn't like processed food, but she can't resist the just-add-water ramen noodle soups. Ditto for the genius No Pudge Fudge, a baking mix that produces single-serving, 100-calorie microwaved brownies in forty seconds.

In terms of dietary trade-offs, Jess doesn't actually make many. As we head for the checkout lane, her trolley contains a bag of split peas, olives, bell peppers, onions, rosemary, parsley, a cantaloupe, brown rice, organic chicken stock, roasted almonds, dried figs, and the brownie and soup mixes. No wonder her skin glows. With the exception of the mixes Jess hasn't bought anything remotely processed.

At the last minute, she remembers that she needs Grana Padano, an Italian cheese, and is dismayed to find that the store doesn't carry it. The Parmigiano on display for $17.99 (£11) a pound is similar, but it looks dried out. She takes a small piece anyway. "It's so expensive," says Jess. "But I'm just buying it because I'm ready to get in line. I need it, and I don't have time to go anywhere else. It's the same old trade-off."

After we part, I think about how Jess shops and what diet lessons might be drawn from her approach. One thing that strikes me is that she doesn't use a list. When I ask her about that, she tells me she mentally keeps track of what staples she needs. As for meat, fruits, and vegetables, she just looks for whatever seems freshest. At the beginning of our expedition, for example, she wanted Brussels sprouts; she described how she would prepare them and expressed regret that her family doesn't like them as much as she does. Instead, she got swept up by some luscious-looking jacket broccoli from Pennsylvania and completely forgot about her Brussels sprouts plans.

For the Manhattan Diet, it's essential to shop this way. You're not only getting what's fresh and so has the most vitamins, you're also getting what appeals to you, which makes dinner more enjoyable. I can hear the hand-wringing now: but how would I cook jacket broccoli? Is it different from regular broccoli? What other ingredients do I need? What does it go with?

I have a solution to all that angst, and it is roasting. I roast everything: broccoli, carrots, cauliflower, green beans, squash, and even kale, which comes out crumbly, crisp, and delicious. That way I know all I need is olive oil and salt and a functioning oven. Jess says she does the same. It's also fast: twenty minutes at 200°C/gas mark 6 for pretty much everything, and you've got a beautiful dish.

The catch is that you have to be an ingredient junkie and care about what you're eating—a lot. I definitely do. Show me a beautiful basket of baby artichokes or perfectly ripe figs, and I will switch dinner plans on a dime. Living with Cesare, I've gotten some coaching, practice, and hand-holding in this area. Cesare will inhale pretty much anything I put in front of him, but he won't stand for mortadella that's been in the refrigerator more than a day or Parmigiano that was cut from a wheel a week earlier.

In the last twenty years, he has trained me to his standards—or spoiled me, however you want to view it. He is also a fantastic supplier. Anytime I want, I can pop by his restaurant to pick up some sheep's milk cheese wrapped in straw, prosciutto from Parma that's been aged three years, or the greatest gift of all, Antinori Peppoli olive oil. In the last few weeks, I've been getting grenade-sized balls of steamed organic broccoli from a farm he works with in Sullivan County. My job has been reduced to sautéing it with a little garlic, dried chilli flakes, and olive oil. It's dreamy.

Not everyone lives with a Cesare, of course. But here, even those who don't will travel miles—schlepping crosstown, uptown, and downtown to obtain the newest, best, or just a favourite speciality item. My friend Janet Ungless, a magazine editor, often takes the bus from the East Side to the Fairway at 74th Street and Broadway because she likes its hummus and its ginger-carrot soup. It's an hour out of her way, but she says it's worth it. Theresa Passarelli, an Upper West Side mom I know, travels fifty blocks south to the Chelsea Market to get the cut of beef she likes for her family. If you're not familiar with Manhattan geography, that's the equivalent of flying from Des Moines to St. Louis for a rack of ribs.

And if the items cost more, so be it. Most of my shoppers would rather have the $11.59 (£7) bottle of organic maple syrup and eke out a tablespoon at a time than buy the cheaper $4.59 (£3) version made with maple flavouring. No contest. I'm not talking about a tiny minority here. Among Manhattan's food literati, two-thirds say they're willing to pay more for organic items or items grown or produced locally, according to a recent Zagat's survey. Even more respondents said it was important to shop for those types of products.

It's a very European way to consume: better a little of something great than a lot of something mediocre. It's not exactly the American way, but it's helpful when you're thinking about retraining your food brain. It goes hand in hand with shopping daily or every other day, which is not uncommon here, either. I didn't interview anyone who does a single mega grocery run per week. In part, that has to do with kitchen size. There just isn't room to stock up on seven days' worth of milk, fruit, and other staples. The fact that most New Yorkers don't have cars, of course, also plays a role—and even those who do don't want to drive just to get groceries. But a lot of it is just temperament. People shop more often because they want their ingredients to be super fresh.

Theresa Passarelli works part-time in her family's commercial property business, and as far as I can tell, she spends the rest of the time grocery shopping and cooking. Like me, she's had high standards drilled into her. Back before "farm to table" was a cliché, Theresa was prepped by her Italian immigrant parents. In their Brooklyn home, picking salad didn't mean choosing between mixed leaves and lettuce. It literally meant finding a field with dandelion stalks and cutting enough to fill a big bowl. When Theresa's dad would bring home a case of fresh figs, she and her siblings cheered. When the family members wanted a roasted chicken, they went to their grandmother's basement, where she raised chickens. "We'd name them, and then they'd be dinner," says Theresa.

Theresa graduated from culinary school, but she could easily have gone the other way and rebelled against all the time and effort it takes to constantly shop and cook. Instead, each week she plans the shopping equivalent of the invasion of Normandy. It's an every-other-day schedule, involving excursions to Whole Foods (for fruit and vegetables), Zabar's (for bread and the store-brand olive oil), Fairway (for staples, including meat) and H&H (for bagels). At least one of those Fairway trips happens on a Thursday morning so she can be sure to get a pack of D'Artagnan turkey mince, which sells out quickly.

She tells me that she shops in order to be in control of what she eats. "Going to different stores is important to me," she adds. "I can tell how food has been handled."

On a Wednesday afternoon while our daughters were in school, Theresa gave me a tour of her kitchen. It was big, by New York standards, about ten feet by fifteen feet, with a pantry that was stocked deep and wide. Lined up like library books were boxes of wholewheat pasta: penne, shells, orecchiette, elbows. She had five different types of canned beans as well as canned tomatoes, chicken stock, maple syrup, brown rice, and white flour. Everything was organic. She's a supermarket owner's dream customer, I thought. In her freezer was chicken stock made from scratch, which she had cooked on a rainy day using chicken parts she'd saved. There were also packs of steak and the organic turkey mince she likes so much.

I recognize Theresa as a fellow brand loyalist, one of those people who after years of trial and error have hit upon the products they think are the best, and they have little patience for store managers, other shoppers, or friends who try to convince them otherwise. In the course of my research, I met quite a few others. Kim Shapiro, who works as an administrator for a hedge fund, scrutinizes pasta sauce labels to make sure the tomatoes used are San Marzano. She has been lobbying Fresh Direct, an online grocer in the metropolitan area, to carry the brand of cottage cheese she likes, Friendship Pot-Style 2% Cottage Cheese. (To no avail; she buys it instead at a grocery near her East Side apartment.) Debi Wisch, the jewellery entrepreneur, is attached to See's lollipops, but they're not sold in New York, so she has them shipped from California.

Theresa has waged battles with managers over everything from the right coffee beans to skirt steaks. Recently, when the five-dollar-a-pound (£6/kg) organic D'Artagnan chickens she likes disappeared from Fairway's poultry counter, she called to complain, only to be told that the store had switched to another purveyor because the D'Artagnan variety was too pricey. This line of reasoning drives her crazy. "I said, 'Pass the price on to the consumer!'" It's not about the price, it's about quality, she says. A roasted, ready-to-eat chicken costs half as much, but it's not as good as the one she makes. She pulls a roasted bird out of the refrigerator to illustrate. "Look. Here's my chicken," she says, squeezing a piece of breast meat between her fingers. It's still moist.

I enjoy observing food warriors in the field, and a great place to start is Eataly, the fifty-thousand-square-foot grocery and restaurant hall on lower Fifth Avenue. Mario Batali and Joe Bastianich are partners there, along with a businessman from Turin, and their idea was to bring the best of Italian groceries and eating under one roof. Eataly is vast and dazzling and packed all day long. I went twice within a few weeks of the opening, and the line was literally out the door—for a grocery store!

At eleven on a Saturday night, Manhattanites with cashmere sweaters tossed over their shoulders and grocery baskets slung over one arm were cruising the aisles for paccheri, anchovies, and marinated artichokes. On a Sunday evening at six a few weeks later, it was the same deal: beautiful people shopping for beautiful food. The dry pasta section alone is double the size of your average 7-Eleven. The fruit and vegetable area looks like a Renaissance still life, with Swiss chard, carrots, and onions too beautiful to handle, let alone mince and sauté. Eataly is carrying Cesare's salumi, and he tells me they are selling seventy whole prosciutti a week. Ten hog legs a day! I bet in Orlando, where I grew up, they don't sell that much prosciutto in six months.

Of course, Eataly exists only in Manhattan. Mario and Joe and their partner would never have opened such a place if it weren't for

Theresa, Debi, Kim, and the thousands like them who shop haute Italian. I think again of Orlando. There are about two million people living there, and the closest thing to an Eataly is Whole Foods. In metropolitan Orlando and the surrounding suburbs, there are two of these stores. In Manhattan, with about half a million fewer people, there are seven Whole Foods, not to mention the gazillion other upscale markets here.

The last time I visited, I went with my dad to the Publix, where he shops. Publix is one of the city's more popular grocery chains, and the company operates more than a thousand stores in the South, many in the fifty-thousand-square-foot range. The Maitland Publix, at Highway 17/92 and Horatio Avenue, is one of the smaller locations, at about thirty thousand square feet. If you think of grocery stores as a reflection of the population they serve, the Publix layout says everything. Of the thirty thousand square feet, only a corner—I estimated it to be five hundred square feet—is devoted to fresh produce.

The Manhattan equivalent of that Publix would be a smallish Food Emporium, like the one on 92nd Street and Broadway. That store looks to be about fifty-five hundred square feet, but the fruit and vegetable section is nearly four hundred square feet. Percentagewise, that's more than four times as much space devoted to fresh produce. Meanwhile, the Food Emporium's fruit and vegetable aisle in late summer looks like a farmers' market. On one Sunday afternoon, there were eleven different types of tomatoes, including heirloom, hothouse, Kumato, grape (two kinds), and cherry. There were as many varieties of bagged leafy greens as there were crisps a few aisles over, including rocket (three kinds), radicchio, pak choi, and Swiss chard.

At the Publix in Orlando, at the same time of year, there was a big variety of lettuce, but only seven heads of broccoli, six packs of Brussels sprouts, and three packs of courgette. There was a twelve-foot case of organic produce with five types of tomatoes and eight varieties of conventional apples. Meanwhile, the store seemed to be promoting fruit that is precut or in bags. Trays of sliced apples and grapes came with a caramel dip. There were no fresh figs, blueberries, or raspberries.

I left the store thinking that Manhattanites don't dip their grapes or their apples in caramel. Manhattan Dieters eat their leafy greens and their orange and yellow vegetables—and their blues and purples and whites and reds. I'm assuming that the law of supply and demand applies to the produce section, which means that New Yorkers demand a lot of fruits and vegetables. Why isn't that true in Orlando?

Can it all be explained away by money? Well, a little bit. There's certainly more of it in Manhattan, and people are willing to spend a lot on their groceries. Although the weekly food bill for a family of four in the U.S. averages between $150 (£90) and $300 (£135), organic-, locavore-, and gourmet-obsessed Manhattan Dieters go much higher. Theresa gave me her receipt from one trip to Fairway. It was $59.41 (£36.50) for sixteen items, all fruits and vegetables except for one bag of $1.99 (£1.20) rice-and-corn-based snack food. Extrapolating from that bill, I put her weekly grocery tab for three at between $250 (£150) and $300 (£180). I spoke to a woman with three kids who spends $500 (£300) *a week*.

Granted, some of this is just because it is more expensive to live in the Big Apple. According to a CNN.com cost-of-living calculator, groceries in New York City are 76 percent pricier than groceries in Buffalo. A Starbucks latte here is $3.75 (£2.30), whereas in Orlando it's $3.35 (£2). And regardless of where you live, eating healthy just costs more. One study I read estimated that a junky, calorie-dense diet costs $3.52 (£2.20) a day, whereas a healthy, low-calorie diet is $36.32 (£22.30) a day. I said before that Manhattan women were willing to pay almost anything for their favourite things, such as artisanal bacon or their bags of frozen organic edamame. But I was overstating. That people spend crazy amounts on their favourite foods isn't in dispute. But Manhattanites count their pennies, too.

Let's take a look at Kimberly Shapiro's shopping trolley.

Married with two young boys, Kim has two grocery priorities: health and price. She does not believe that processed foods are by definition evil. She's one of those ingredient warriors who will go to all lengths to get the brands she likes best. If those brands happen to be made in a plant in Northfield, Illinios (home to Kraft, in case you're wondering), so be it. I would describe her as a conscientious shopper, not a dogmatic one. Among other things, she finds organic produce awful—"it wilts," she says—and dieting a waste of time. "It's all common sense. You eat less, exercise more."

We are sitting at Kim's granite-topped kitchen table on the East Side. She is deep in online shopping, placing her weekly Fresh Direct order. Clicking through the site, Kim snaps up, with equal conviction, items like wild coho salmon fillets and Danimals Crush Cup yogurt (drinkable yogurt aimed at kids that comes in a soft plastic container that you have to crush in your hand before you can drink it), wholewheat pasta and Fat-Free French Vanilla Coffee-Mate.

She tells me that high cholesterol runs in her family and that her husband watches his weight. So her shopping priority is choosing items that will help on those fronts. She likes a brand of butter that contains rapeseed oil, for example, because it has four grams of saturated fat versus eleven in the regular butter, and Popchips, a variation on the crisps that has four grams of fat per one-ounce serving, compared to ten grams of fat for an ounce of other regular brands. She's not averse to time-savers, like partially baked sourdough rolls, and she buys 90-calorie Quaker Oats bars, also low in fat.

Mostly, it seems, Kim loves a good sale. You can hear it in her running commentary on her various purchases. Those Danimals Crush Cups are often criticized by children's health advocates as "liquid candy" for their high sugar content (a tablespoon in each portion according to some food blogs), but Kim's two sons love them, and when she spots them on her screen, she clicks immediately. "You open it, you crush it; you drink it. You don't need a spoon or a glass. It's genius, and it's on sale for $1.99 (£1.20). Even better."

Kim passes on strawberries; she'd like to buy them, but not at this price. She loves Brussels sprouts, but not at $4.99 (£3) a bag; scallops at $19.99 a pound (£25/kg) prompt her to roll her eyes. "Forget that," she snorts. When she spots wild coho salmon on sale for $11.99 a pound (£15/kg) instead of $15.99 a pound (£20/kg), however, Kim grabs the mouse and clicks into action. "This is the perfect time to buy it. I'll freeze it."

Until recently, Kim did all of her grocery shopping in person. But last year, when her father passed away, she didn't have the energy to deal with the lines and the crowds, so she switched to Fresh Direct. Because of people like Kim, the company has become something of a local phenomenon, surviving (even thriving) when other online grocers have failed. Fresh Direct's signature vans, splashed with a leafy orange and green logo, are fixtures on the streets of Manhattan, and the company's customers swear by its next-day delivery. "Sometimes the quality is worse. But if you buy something that is awful and you e-mail them, they will give you a credit," Kim tells me.

Kim grew up in Queens in a family in which healthy eating was emphasized. Fizzy drinks and sugary cereals weren't allowed in the house, and her father, a physician, insisted that the family have salad every day. She never had weight issues, but when she went to college and started eating pizza and drinking beer late at night, she gained almost two stone. As she shed that weight, she became more conscious of nutrition and eating well, and today, at age forty-three, she weighs between nine stone four pounds and nine stone nine pounds, less than she did in high school.

Her attitude to food now is very no-nonsense. She watches herself at home, but if she is at a restaurant known for lasagne, she'll order the lasagne—and finish it. As she reviews her Fresh Direct order, she notes how many items she got for $187.21 (£115). "There's nothing in here that isn't healthy," she says. "I'm not so calorie conscious, but I want to make sure I get all the food groups in me—the omega-3s, the B12s," she says.

One reason the Manhattan Dieter's ingredient radar is so finely tuned is that it goes with her type A personality. If you buy ingredients and cook food yourself, you know exactly what is going into a dish. There's no guessing about the fat content, the calories, the carbs, or any other aspect of a meal's nutritional value. Dietitians, in fact, encourage their patients to eat more home-cooked meals for that very reason: it eliminates the guesswork.

Equally important is that shopping gives eaters control over their pantries. Chocolate tea cakes—yes or no? Almonds—smoked, salted, or raw? Low-fat sour cream or the full-fat version? Again and again, Manhattanites ban foods from their pantries simply because they pose too much temptation. You name it, they've done away with it: peanut butter, white sugar, cereal, dinner rolls, butter, chocolate bars, ice cream, ready-made cupcake frosting, biscuits, crackers.

"I don't want the extra food in there, because I will eat it," says Nina Kaminer, the owner of Nike Communications, a public relations firm. "It's neurotic behavior," she says, but she can't help herself. It's why she shops for groceries daily or every other day and why her refrigerator is mostly empty—it gives her a sense of satisfaction. "It's like I'm so well-behaved. I will only have this amount of food."

There is also an element of show-off behaviour here. Want the fantastic-mother imprimatur? With a simple thirty-minute spin through the organics aisle, a mom can show her commitment to the environment and to the health of her children (and to her own ego). You can make all of your meals from scratch or swear completely off white sugar or processed foods—it's the shopping high road, easy to take if you've got the cash, the time, the fortitude, and the personality.

In my research, I ran into the tidal wave of research about obesity and diabetes and the divide between the healthy and well-heeled and the poor. I can't avoid acknowledging the issue, because it makes me feel shallow and ridiculous to write about shopping for five-dollar-a-pound (£6/kg) organic chicken when so many people can't afford to spend five dollars (£3) a day on food for their families.

But that's really another book altogether. My only observation is that there's been a shift in the last few years, so that most of the research now blames obesity on the cost and lack of availability of healthy food. In the past, the blame was more along the lines of "you're fat because you don't have self control." The truth may lie somewhere in between, but in talking to Manhattanites, I found that old opinions die hard. Pretty much everyone I interviewed summed up their dieting strategy as follows: eat less. Exercise more. Don't buy food you shouldn't eat. Read your labels. It's one of the Michael Pollan credos: eat food, just less of it.

What's the message you should take away from all this? What's your grocery priority? Is it convenience? Organic food? Price? You might not have the motivation of Theresa Passarelli to hit four grocery stores in a day to secure the freshest ingredients for your turkey tacos. But you might want to find a good organic food company and place an order with them.

I remember when Cesare first moved to Manhattan and couldn't get the dishes he was cooking to come out exactly as they'd been in Italy. He realized pretty quickly it was the ingredients. The courgettes, tomatoes, olive oil, whatever, aren't the same here as they are there. The resulting tomato sauce, timbale, or whatever it was he was making didn't come out the same. So he figured out how to use the ingredients he had to produce the food he wanted.

Here are some of the diet foods my diary keepers said they keep in their refrigerators and pantries:

Almonds

Pickled ginger (no calories!)

Tinned tuna (Drain, break over a bowl of lettuce, and dinner is done.)

Boiled egg whites (Keep bowls of them handy in the refrigerator for a quick kick of protein.)

Lean, organic steak (You can buy this already marinated; just sear on both sides and eat.)

No-butter butter spray (In the UK, Frylight Better Than Butter oil spray is a good option.)

Low-fat salad dressing sprays

Weight Watchers pizza (not organic, but pretty good for frozen pizza)

Beans (chickpeas, cannellini, kidney. They are filling, full of fibre, and low in fat. Toss them into salads, or make a bean salad with a teaspoon of good olive oil and vinegar.)

Fat-free vanilla yogurt

Greek-style yogurt

Agave syrup (healthier than honey)

Dairy-free "ice cream" sandwiches and bars—a lifesaver in the summer)

Dried cherries, almonds, and tamari, a mix sold at a store where one of my interviewees volunteers (You can make it at home with soy.)

Frozen grapes

Veggie burgers or sausages (which kids love with mustard or ketchup)

Skinny Cow ice creams

High-fibre cake bars

Fruit and nut bars (such as Nakd)

Low-fat rice pudding

Low-fat cereals (such as Cheerios, Shredded Wheat and Special K)

Porridge (the real rolled oats kind, not the instant)

Low-fat fudge brownie mix (Add 1 tablespoon of yogurt to 2 tablespoons of the fudge mix, and you've got a low-calorie, microwaved brownie in forty seconds.)

Manhattan Diet Secrets

- *Shop around.* Find a store that reflects the way that you want to eat and that actually works at stocking healthy, wholesome ingredients. The market doesn't have to be organic, it just has to have a wide selection of fruits and vegetables; fresh poultry, other meats, and fish; and real cheese, not processed "cheese food" or vac-packed bars of cheddar with the shelf life of carbon-14.

- *Garbage in, garbage out.* Don't buy crappy ingredients. It defeats the purpose. I don't mean that you must eat lobster and not tilapia. Tilapia is a pretty tasty fish. But checkout-counter sushi is wrong. So are apples with caramel dip. Take the time to learn about food and how to prepare it. Look for what's fresh and seasonal.

- *Learn to read—labels, that is.* You know the drill: avoid products with additives you can't pronounce and foods whose first five ingredients include corn syrup, high-fructose corn syrup, cellulose gum, and caramel colour. Don't be misled by phrases like "trans fat–free" and "all natural." Arsenic is all natural. You don't want that in your breakfast cereal. Most chocolate tea cakes, cheesy crackers, and microwave popcorn contain zero trans fats, but they're loaded with other stuff you want to avoid.

- *Shop early, shop often.* The fresher your ingredients, the more nutrients they retain. It's pretty simple, and it's also why it's preferable to buy broccoli in the summer from a local farmer who picked it the day before selling it at the farmers' market. The broccoli shipped in from California that costs half the price will have been picked a week or more before it gets to the grocery store, where it sits for a few days more before you buy it. And you know how long stuff sits in your fridge.

- *Fat is your friend.* I encourage you to avoid foods that have had the fat zapped out of them or that are made to be low-fat from the get-go. I happen to love fat-free Greek yogurt, but full-fat foods make you feel fuller and more satisfied. Packaged diet foods like fat-free cookies or low-fat salad dressing make you fatter. If you don't believe me, read Michael Pollan.

5

Walk the Walk, Talk the Talk

How We Exercise

I am strapped onto a stationary bicycle at Soul Cycle on the Upper East Side. The music is blaring. The instructor is barking. The other students are pedalling. I am a yoga girl, and I also run. I am completely out of my element.

Yet I am here because I've been told that Stacey Griffith, today's teacher—the one with surfer chick arms, a yellow bandanna, and purple satin trainers—is a Fitness Goddess. Rather, she is the Fitness Goddess of the moment, a Lady Gaga for the Lululemon Athletica crowd. Stacey used to ply her trade on the other coast but was lured to Manhattan a few years ago by the founders of the studio. My impression is that the deal has worked out for everyone:

Stacey, who's become a local star; her bosses, who've cashed in on her success; and the students, who worship at Stacey's feet.

Before her followers know what they want from a workout, Stacey is there, anticipating every pedal, curl, and press. From the looks of it, I'd say that what those followers want is a body mass index under 18 with ripped abs and rock-hard pecs, and from the looks of it, I'd say that Stacey is doing her job pretty well. My bike happens to be parked behind that of a very trim Lulu Johnson, designer Betsy Johnson's daughter and a fixture on the gossip pages. I hear Lulu is a regular. Checking out the room, I don't spot any other celebrities, although I've read that everyone from Katie Couric to model Hana Soukupova works out here. If there is more than an ounce of superfluous body fat in the room, it's all on me.

Class has just started, but I'm already over the experience. It took me two weeks just to reserve a bike. That's par for the course. As soon as something catches on in Manhattan, it's impossible to get in on the action. You've got to know someone, pay someone, or otherwise divine the magic password. My friend Ali has shared the Soul Cycle secret with me. You don't just click willy-nilly around the website until you find a class with Stacey. I tried that. All of her classes are full—always. The trick, Ali tells me, is to log in on Monday exactly at noon and sign up at the time and location you want for the coming week. And be fast.

This image pops into my head: it's 11:45 a.m. on Monday morning, and women up and down Manhattan, all wearing form-fitting workout togs, are poised at their laptops. Hand on trackbar, each is clicking anxiously, hoping to get a spot first. I have slipped in by default. I made a waiting list, then moved up, and finally got a call from the studio with the news I'd made the cut.

With all of the pumping up and down, sideways, and back and forth, this class isn't for me. But the women in the class are driven. They are serious. I can see it, even in the darkened room with strobe lights flashing. Are they the exception or the rule when it comes to exercise? I can't help but wonder, and afterwards, I ask Stacey about her regulars. She tells me that she calls them her "ninja mommies," a phrase I love. "They're in it to win it," she adds.

Stacey talks a little like a motivational guru, coming out with things like "Go to your sexiest place!" and "This is your time!" through her headset. Some of her students are so hooked, she tells me, they take back-to-back 9:30 and 10:30 a.m. sessions. I check Soul Cycle's website and read that a single class burns off about 500 calories. That means that some of my morning's classmates will have vaporized 1,000 calories before noon. The Food and Drug Administration's daily recommended calorie allowance is 2,000, so they've already burned off half a day's eating. I'm in awe.

It's Manhattan, Stacey says. Normal. "When I taught in L.A., it was to actors and models and the unemployed, and they were all into their own rides. Here, it's 95 percent mommies. They take it seriously. It's like the difference between fans of the Lakers and fans of the Knicks." Manhattanites are hardcore.

Work hard, play hard, work out harder. It sounds like a Nike ad. But that's the Manhattan drill. There are all sorts of reasons you might think we don't get exercise here: limited park space, ridiculously high gym fees, fewer swimming pools per capita than pretty much any city in the United States. Yet Manhattanites, in the neighbourhood of 8 percent obesity rates and average household incomes of $120,000 (£75,000) and higher, are fitness fiends. It goes hand in hand with why we diet and eat well: everyone else does. It's good for you. It will make you live longer, reduce stress, release pheromones, and all of the other things exercise is supposed to do.

No matter how crazy busy Manhattan women are, they figure a way to sneak exercise into their day. I've got friends who bike to work. Some only take stairs, never elevators. One mom I know scooters two miles every morning to take her kids to school.

But those are the exceptions. Mostly women here exercise in the traditional way, the same way women do everywhere: in a gym, running, playing a sport, or working with a trainer. They do yoga, cardio, weight lifting, core building, or strength training; they run, or they play tennis. Some are into pole dancing, others into hula hooping or belly dancing. There's also boxing and elliptical biking. You name it, New Yorkers do it.

A big reason is the fluke of topography that affects how Manhattanites eat and live. I've talked about this already, but you can't get away from it. The fact that apartments here are smushed together cheek by jowl with delis, office buildings, cinemas, and drugstores informs almost everything people do. Out in Iowa or Ohio, life is spread out. You need a carton of milk, you get in the car and go buy it. Here you take a ten-minute walk to the deli.

There is a scene in the movie *L.A. Story* in which Steve Martin gets into his car, drives twenty feet to a neighbour's house, and gets out. I remember it because it was funny. But I also remember it because in the cinema where I saw it, the laughter was almost reflexive, with all of the Manhattanites reacting in smug unison: suckers! How can they live like that?

If Los Angelenos are in love with their cars, New Yorkers are all about sensible footwear. Although there is no shortage of glittery shoe boutiques, there are entire women's shoe stores without a single stiletto or even kitten heel; the stock is instead made entirely of sturdy shoes and boots that are designed for walking three miles a day and more. But because walking is so much a part of daily life, no one consciously thinks about it or even considers it actual exercise.

It's like eating a cookie standing up, except it's the opposite. Because you don't think about the walking, the calories you burn scarcely register as exercise. The typical New Yorker logs about 1.2 miles a day just walking to and from the bus or subway. In a research project in Charlotte, North Carolina, commuters who added that mileage to their daily routine for six months lost an average of 1.18 BMI points. Ladies, lace up your trainers! If you're five feet five and ten stone ten pounds, and you start walking 1.2 miles a day for six months, like the Charlotte commuters, you could slim down by six and a half pounds.

And walking is just the first step, so to speak, for fit Manhattanites. All of that sidewalk time translates into training. In better shape from the get-go, walking New Yorkers are prepped for other, more strenuous exercise routines. It is a hand-in-glove romance that has been going on for decades, and it partly accounts for the high percentage of gyms here: 226, or one for every sixty-six hundred or so residents, according to the International Health, Racquet, and Sports Club Association. Metropolitan Chicago has 479 member clubs, one for about every twenty thousand locals.

The benefits of all the walking and exercising that Manhattanites do show up in longevity studies. A New Yorker born in 2004 can now expect to live 78.6 years, nine months longer than the average American. The life expectancy of New Yorkers is increasing at a rate faster than that of most of the rest of the country, too. Since 1990, the average American has added only about 2.5 years to her life, but New Yorkers have added 6.2 years to theirs—more than double! Amazing, isn't it? Living in Manhattan is like living in a gym. It's just good for you.

There *are* those here who don't work out, but in my circle they're the minority. You go to the gym because your friends do, because everyone talks about their trainers and gym fees and hamstrings, and you don't think you have a choice. It's identity. I've been doing yoga for about twelve years. I used to practise an arduous kind called Ashtanga that leaves you (or at least left me) with perilously tender knees and a very sore lower back. But I powered through, and at my most obsessive, I was taking three two-hour classes a week. Eventually I turned to more gentle forms of yoga, and over the years, my attendance dwindled to just one class a week.

That was until my friend Janet said something along the lines of "You wuss! You can't stay in shape going to yoga once a week." I was so irritated, and I remember dismissing her with a roll of my eyes. Like, what do you know? Without ever really acknowledging that she was right, I started running, eventually building up to three or four times a week, in addition to doing yoga.

So now I'm where I should be, exercisewise. Basically, I caved in to my friend's expectation. She goaded; I reacted. It's part of the social contract. And it does give me an identity of sorts. I'm not a Spinner (too East Side), not a weight lifter (too boring), and not a private-trainer addict (too expensive). I don't even like going to a fancy gym (too corporate). Yoga and running fit me just right. Those are my issues, of course, and everyone has her own.

The jockeying and the mind games are all part of a whole, says Dalton Conley, the dean of New York University's Department of Sociology. Where you work out, like where you shop for groceries, is a signifier. "It's not the Harvard Club, but it is a status symbol," he says.

In spite of New Yorkers' fitness prowess, somewhere along the line we somehow got a bad rap as exercise wimps. Maybe it has to do with the declining fortune of the Knicks. Or George Steinbrenner, the now-deceased Yankee boss. Why not? He had as much to do with it as anyone else—that is, nothing at all. It's just a bunch of Manhattan bashing. It sells magazines, Google ads, or whatever attracts advertisers these days.

. . . .

How They Diet

HELENA CHRISTENSEN

The supermodel, who posed in the buff (except for trainers) in a Reebok ad at age forty-one, is a cheese addict, and she says she's even toyed with the idea of getting a cheese tattoo on her shoulder. She eats lots of different foods in five small meals a day. She also works out like crazy: boxing, running, and dancing.

. . . .

A few years ago, *Men's Fitness* ranked the Big Apple the fifth fattest city in the United States. The magazine faulted the city for its lack of golf courses and tennis courts. It slapped the city on the wrist for not enough fitness centres and sports stores. It gave New Yorkers a D+ for participation and an F+ for city recreational facilities. *Men's Fitness* isn't alone. Over the years, New York has popped up on other media city lists for least fit, unhealthiest, or unhappiest.

Hogwash! The editors gave Manhattan a B– on motivation, for God's sake! What does *Men's Fitness* know? Have its editors been to Barbara Becker's apartment at 7:15 on a typical school morning? Clearly not. Barbara is a friend of my friend Oona, who touts Barbara as a paragon of fitness, someone who works out almost every day. Once we start talking, I see that Oona has pretty much nailed it.

Barbara is the quintessential busy type who knows how to squeeze anything into her schedule. That's no easy task when you've got four kids and a big job. Barbara is forty-six years old, five feet five, and eight stone nine pounds. Her kids range from four to eleven years old. She is a lawyer with a national firm and does securities work. Barbara travels for her job and also does work dinners and school events. She lives with her husband and kids on the Upper West Side. Three of their children go to a private school with two locations across Central Park on the East Side, about a mile away.

That's pretty daunting, from an exercise point of view. Who has the time? Who has the energy? Yet here's what happens every morning at the Becker household. At 7:15, Barbara, Barbara's husband, and all four kids strap on safety helmets, pull out their Razor scooters, and begin their morning journey. The first stop is the lower school, where one child is dropped off. That's about a twenty-minute ride across town. By 7:45, the entourage has scooted north about three-quarters of a mile to where the upper school is located. Two more kids get dropped off there.

After the second group is settled in, Barbara parks her Razor in a designated spot and walks to her gym, aiming to arrive by 8 a.m. She works out for half an hour to forty-five minutes, then makes her way to the office (via subway) in Midtown. Her husband, meanwhile, returns to the West Side by scooter with the four-year-old and drops that child off at preschool. When Barbara picks up her kids in the afternoon, she starts by retrieving the scooter and then does a reverse commute. She's not just committed to exercise, she's addicted to it. "That's how we build in activity," says Barbara, "For us, walking is too slow."

I admit, you've got to be a bit of a nut to scoot around the city delivering your children to school in the morning just to squeeze in some exercise. But it's the right kind of nuttiness. It's the nuttiness that says that in spite of the difficulties, you've made a decision to keep fit and you're going to stick to it. The method doesn't have to be so extreme. It could just be doing fifteen minutes of stretches at home in the morning—or doing sit-ups, or doing whatever.

The key word is *doing*. If Barbara can figure out a way to work out every day, so can anyone. That's my theory, anyway. People exercise against the odds all over the place: Phoenix, Atlanta, St. Louis, even Corpus Christi—which has been ranked as *the* fattest city in the country by *Men's Health*. It's the making-lemonade-from-lemons approach.

Look at the park situation in Manhattan. It's hard to argue with the fact that New York City as a whole doesn't have as much open space as, for instance, Los Angeles. Griffith Park, L.A.'s most famous park, is an enormous 4,210 acres northwest of the city's downtown area. Manhattan's biggest park is Central Park, at just 843 acres, smack in the middle of the island. But guess what? Proportionately, New York is way ahead. Central Park accounts for 6 percent of Manhattan's land mass, whereas Griffith Park is less than 2 percent of L.A. proper.

What's more, Central Park's location is key. Apparently, we in Manhattan are more likely to use our parks than our counterparts in L.A. are, because ours are so accessible. In fact, when the RAND Corporation looked at a handful of L.A. parks, it found that the majority of people who frequented any given park lived no more than a quarter of a mile away. Only 13 percent of the people using the park had come from more than a mile away.

The mere fact of geography, that we are all crammed in together, means it's actually easier to do things like run, play in parks, or go to yoga or a gym. Whereas some studies show that Americans don't exercise because they don't have the motivation, Manhattanites say they exercise because they don't have an excuse not to. Every neighbourhood has a New York Sports Club, an Equinox, an indy yoga studio, or a Crunch, and sometimes multiples. In the Midtown mile between 33rd and 54th Streets, there are five Equinoxes alone.

"I don't have to jump in a car and drive forty-five minutes to my exercise class," says Nancy Trent, a longtime New Yorker who lives in SoHo, a neighbourhood known more for loft apartments, art galleries, and boutiques than for sweaty workouts. Trent's loft, in fact, is just a short stroll from both gyms she frequents—yes, she belongs to two—as well as from her office, a public relations firm that she owns. Who needs to schlep to exercise?

Because it's so easy to reach her gym, because exercise calms her down, and because she's a bit obsessed, Nancy works out every day. She starts at seven in the morning, with either an hour-long Core Fusion class at Exhale (an intense, athletic routine) or a ninety-minute Bikram yoga class, which is done in a 35° to 40°C degree studio. Bikram is supposed to detoxify the body and aid everything from the circulatory system to the relief of lower back pain.

"I don't work out for my body. I work out for my brain," the PR executive tells me. "I have a stressful job. Part of my job description is being hysterical *and* in a good mood. I have to be upbeat. One way for me to be upbeat is to exercise." Nancy adds that she sees the two types of exercise as complementing each other: Core Fusion is the hard work, Bikram is what she calls "a vacation. You're exhausted, but out of that comes great energy and strength."

I have to interject here that I took a Core Fusion class at Exhale a few years ago. I did it at the urging of my pal Janet, the same one who more recently shamed me into exercising more often. That first time, she was less successful. The class reminded me of what used to be called calisthenics before marketers got their hands on fitness lingo and started coming up with catchy names for everything. It had lots of repetitions of leg lifts, squats, and what Jane Fonda dubbed "going for the burn."

After the Core Fusion class, my butt burned, my triceps burned, my everything burned. I just didn't care about being in that kind of shape. It wasn't for the faint of heart (or, at thirty-five dollars (£3) a class, the weak of pocket), and the fact that Nancy does this every other day of her life signals that she is way out of my league. That she does it on alternating days with Bikram signals that she is probably out of most sane people's exercise league.

Another tip-off in that regard: while we are chatting, Nancy tells me that she is into "compression garments" as a weight-loss aid. These are girdle-like items that are supposed to help you slim down because they squeeze your muscles all day long, theoretically helping you burn more calories. "I'm sort of exercising while I'm talking to you," she says.

Still, to her credit, Nancy allows that working out as much as she does isn't always fun. "If you ask me what time it is at any point during the day, I never know," she says. "In Bikram I always know what time it is." Her favourite part of class is the *shavasana*, or corpse pose, when students lie still on their backs at the end of class to rest. Because many of Nancy's clients are in the spa or health industries, staying in shape goes with the territory. She needs to look good to promote herself and her brands. It's part of her daily life, her job.

Where'd You Get Those Abs?

The first step in getting fit like a Manhattanite is knowing the routines. Here are some locals' favourite workouts.

Exercise: Bikram, or Hot, Yoga

What it is: Ninety minutes of yoga done in a room at a temperature of 35°–40° degrees.

Benefits: Purifies the body's systems and helps with everything from respiratory issues to lower back pain and arthritis.

Who practises it: Nancy Trent, Lady Gaga, Madonna.

Watch out for: Your neighbour's sweat will drip all over you.

Comment: Even on days when the temperature in the city is in the thirties, classes are packed.

Exercise: Kangoo Jumps

What it is: Running in specially designed spring shoes that propel the runner up and down, like a pogo stick. It is an offshoot of the rebounding, or mini-trampoline, craze.

Benefits: Said to provide the aerobic benefits of running without the wear and tear on the joints.

Who practises it: Hyperfit young people who bound together, up and down Manhattan streets, often stopping traffic.

Watch out for: You need to be an exhibitionist. Men Kangoo Jumpers tend to practise the sport sans shirt; women seem to prefer jogging bras, no cover-up.

Comment: I can't vouch for this form of exercise except to say, as a bystander, it's good for a laugh.

Exercise: Bands Spinning

What it is: Spinning classes made even harder. During a class, oversized resistance bands drop from the ceiling so that the students can grab onto them and work out their arms, abs, backs, and chests while they cycle.

Benefits: Adds strengthening exercises to the cardio workout of cycling.

Who practises it: Kelly Ripa, Brooke Shields, and Kyra Sedgwick, as well as lots of other Manhattan celebs. Diehards go for the bands classes.

Watch out for: If you don't have the coordination to stand and bike at the same time, adding resistance bands to the mix could spell trouble.

Comment: The Spinning studio Flywheel Sports equips each bike with a digital display showing the rider's real-time stats. Riders can hook up to a screen and share their RPM with classmates.

Exercise: Boot Camp

What it is: A military-like workout, with obstacle courses, lunges, push-ups, jump squats, and hurdles.

Benefits: A whole-body workout to reduce body fat and body size and to increase strength.

Who practises it: Serious fitness geeks.

Watch out for: It's not just ex-Marines who operate these camps, though many advertise themselves as such. Sometimes it's just very fit young people.

Comment: A six-week platinum wedding package (five days a week) to prepare you for the big day can add up to seven thousand dollars (just under five thousand pounds).

Exercise: Pole Dancing

What it is: Get in shape and release your inner exotic dancer.

Benefits: Strength, agility, and flexibility.

Who practises it: Public relations firm owner Nina Kaminer and actress Sheila Kelley, founder of the S Factor.

Watch out for: Scouts from the Scores strip club. Christina Applegate's pregnant pole-dancing routine on Funnyordie.com won her a ten-thousand-dollar offer from Scores to dance for real.

Comment: "When I leave after two hours, I feel wrung out," says Kaminer. "I have much more strength in my upper arms, my core is tighter, I have more flexibility"—not unlike an exotic dancer. "I just turned fifty and I look pretty good."

Exercise: Physique 57

What it is: A choreographed fifty-seven minutes of work that focuses on the core. Founded by a former Wall Street banker.

Benefits: A sculptured butt.

Who practises it: Kelly Ripa, Emmy Rossum, Parker Posey, Christy Turlington.

Watch out for: The Physique 57 routine is good for strength building and small muscle groups, but you will probably have to get your cardio elsewhere.

Comment: A study Physique 57 conducted with Adelphi University followed thirty-eight women who took four Physique 57 classes per week, four weeks in a row. The women didn't restrict calories (but did eat healthy), and all lost weight. Great marketing tool!

. . . .

If you are grimacing and thinking that exercise as lifestyle sounds like a slogan dreamed up by some marketing executive, you're right. You are what you eat, you are where you shop, and now you are what exercise you do. *Please!* Nevertheless, there is some truth to it. As I was saying before, the exercise you do says something about your personality, and so does the way you integrate exercise into your life. Anna Wintour is a big tennis player. Kelly Ripa does Core Fusion and runs. Christine Baranksi walks a lot and does Pilates. Each regimen fits its subject.

I ran this idea by Elisabeth Halfpapp, the creator of Core Fusion and the founder of Exhale, where I've been doing yoga for three years. Elisabeth has been a figure on the Manhattan exercise scene for decades, and she set it a-twitter when she defected from Lotte Berk, the studio where she taught for many years, to open Exhale. We don't know each other, but so many of the women I've spoken to have recommended her as a source that I gave her a call. She is very gracious and takes fitness very seriously—a little too much, for my taste. But she knows the industry and backs up my "you are what you exercise" theory. Instead of being a means to an end, exercise is something her clients do because they like to, Elisabeth says.

It's an alternative to going to the movies or to a museum or curling up with a book. It's not exercise, it's entertainment. Ten or twenty years ago, I think New Yorkers were more interested just in being skinny. That was the point of working out. But once the yoga revolution took hold, things shifted. People all over the country started doing downward dog, upward dog, twisting themselves every which way to get in shape and in tune with their inner yogis. Once exercise got soul, the door to fitness as a lifestyle choice was opened. On its heels came everything from health bars and work-out-wear boutiques inside gyms to luxury yoga retreats in South America. New Yorkers jumped on the trend, and it stuck.

When I made the rounds in some local gyms, I saw the lifestyle in action. I was pretty dazzled by the setup at the Sports Club/L.A. on the Upper East Side. It's got a boxing studio, a Pilates studio, a sea of elliptical machines and Stairmasters, climbing walls, squash courts, and dozens of daily classes. The club also has two full bas-ketball courts, which are so spacious that teams that come to town to play the Knicks sometimes rent the space for practice. When manager Chris Oehl gave me a tour, he showed me a rooftop terrace set up like a country club, with chaise longues, a barbecue, a bar, and waiter service. On Wednesday nights, he told me, the club shows movies and serves popcorn and wine. It also offers lectures on health, provides childcare, and has a lobby juice bar where you can grab a post-workout smoothie or a snack.

I also checked out Pure, an upscale yoga chain owned by Equinox. Outside each individual studio is the equivalent of a living room, with built-in sofas, squishy pillows, and more magazines than in my dentist's office. It's the yoga studio as a second home. It's a lifestyle! It's synergy!

Of course, if Manhattanites didn't actually like exercise, they wouldn't keep going back to Equinox, Exhale, Pure, or the Sports Club/L.A. Even here, marketing can go only so far. The key is internalizing the message. Lillie Rosenthal, an osteopath who works with members of the New York City Ballet corps, says she always counsels her patients to find an exercise they enjoy. Otherwise they won't do it. The advice is not as obvious as it seems, since many of her clients come to her with aches and pains they've developed from routines that they perform by rote or that are just plain wrong for their body types. In this scenario, Debi Wisch is the *Glamour* "Do"—the girl who gets it right.

You might remember Debi from chapter 3. She owns a designer jewellery business, has a kitchen that looks like an extension of Whole Foods, and eats organic, except when she's serving peanut butter pie or a velvet cake to guests or sneaking a lollipop. Debi is also the one who dropped to the floor during our interview to show me her side plank and push-ups. When I admired her arms, she told me, "They're the same at forty-six as they were at twenty-six." I didn't know her at twenty-six, but at forty-six, she looks pretty darn good.

Debi was raised in Winnipeg, in Manitoba, Canada, and has exercise in her DNA. Her dad and her brothers were all jocks, and she grew up playing tennis and baseball, jogging, and water-skiing. Today, she says, she works out for fun, although I think the Michelle Obama biceps must be a motivation, too. She clearly dabbles in all kinds of exercise, but she is quick to drop things that bore her (weight lifting), are inefficient (yoga), or are just too time-consuming. (Debi was unimpressed by Tracy Anderson, fitness guru to Gwyneth Paltrow. "It's two hours a day, six days a week. I don't want to be like that!" she says.)

Instead, three times a week she hits a Spin class with Stacey at Soul Cycle, and on alternate days she takes boxing at Punch. On Sundays, she takes a two-hour-long walk with her husband, either in Central Park, which is across the street from their Fifth Avenue apartment, or on the beach of their weekend house in the Hamptons. "It's more like a lifestyle thing," Debi tells me. "It's not to stay in shape. If it's not fun, you don't want to do it. Life can be tough. You should enjoy things. Go to the gym and not like it? Why? It's an hour and a half of my time."

I have one last thought about how Manhattanites exercise, and it's not a flattering one. If you've ever been to a gym here, you'll know what I mean. For some reason, all of the city's worst character traits seem to come out in workout facilities: the competition, the backbiting, the striving, the lack of grace. You see it in the fights for mat space in class, in the dirty tricks used to finagle a swim lane, and in the battles to corner the newest elliptical trainer. The gym floor is like a microcosm of dog-eat-dog Wall Street. Maybe it's all the endorphins that get released during a workout; I'm not sure.

The good news is that regardless of what prompts the bad behaviour, it works to the exerciser's advantage. I happened to be talking to my friend Lauren the other day, and she mentioned working out on an elliptical trainer at her gym. Lauren got on the machine next to a woman of similar age and build. Naturally, Lauren tells me, she got competitive. She started wondering how much the woman weighed and how old she was. Then it escalated to "If she's going to a harder level, I'm going to last longer than she does."

Not only did Lauren outperform her unknown competitor, she was proud of herself. When she realized that, she slapped herself on the wrist. "I said, I have to get off the elliptical trainer," and she did. But a little competition never hurt anyone, especially on the gym floor. Be on the lookout for your local Lauren.

Manhattan Diet Secrets

- *Invest in some trainers and start walking.* It is the baseline exercise in Manhattan and readies you for everything that follows. Start small and build up. Then you can run. That's what I did last summer. I started walking half a mile. Then I ran it, then I walked and ran a mile, and then I ran a mile. Now I run three miles three or four times a week.

- *Get competitive.* Forget the "everyone's a winner" mentality. You have to compete. Beat everyone around you at the gym, in yoga class, and on the track.

- *Sneak it in.* Ur-Manhattanite Sarah Jessica Parker says that one of the ways she stays in shape is by taking stairs instead of elevators. She carries her baby instead of using a stroller. I carry my groceries five blocks (about a quarter of a mile) instead of taking a taxi home. Small choices add up.

- *Cross-train.* Look for exercises that combine aerobics with strength training so you get two workouts in one. That's very New York, says Chris Oehl of the Sports Club/L.A., which explains why the gym is offering more classes like Athletic-works and Cardio Sculpt, Rocking Yoga, and Splash Aqua Mix.

- *Have fun.* If you pick an exercise you like, it will seem less like work. What's drearier than an hour in a Steps class if you don't like to dance?

6

The Manhattan Diet
Weight-Loss Plan
How We Got This Way

It's time for the reveal. You know, the turning point in my story, where I move from sharing chatty observations about foodies, Cesare, and juice fasts to the brass tacks of the Manhattan Diet. In other words, this is the part where I hand over the rules you've been waiting for, the practical advice you can cut out and tape to the refrigerator. I've got a few things I want to clarify first. As I've noted earlier, I'm a journalist and a food obsessive. I'm not a dietitian, a chef, or an epidemiologist. I don't have a degree in nutrition. With the exception of having a few sessions with Eric Powell, my genius Ashtanga yoga teacher, I've never used any kind of personal trainer.

But over the course of my adult life, and especially in the last year, I've become a de facto expert on the Manhattan Diet. To achieve that status, I did what journalists do. I talked to a lot of people: health professionals of every stripe, food professionals, exercise pros, academics, and chefs. I shanghaied every fit, slender, toned woman I know into sharing her eating habits: lawyers, nurses, bankers, editors, ad execs, and stay-at-home moms; women with eating issues and those without; women who live on breakfast bars, 24/7 grazers, and three-meal-a-dayers.

As I interviewed these people, I also read studies. I sifted through data. I formed theories. I decided to do more interviews and more reading. Yet I am the first to point out that this is not a scientific or medically proven diet book. It is, however, a deeply reported, anecdotally driven, in-depth chronicle of how a very slim population on a very small island goes about its eating business. In this, it has no peer.

In order to create the Manhattan Diet, I went back to the women I'd been interviewing and asked them to keep food diaries. I asked them to write down every morsel that went into their mouths for a week in the late autumn of 2010. I asked them to note the time of day, the portion size, their thoughts at the time, and any exercise they might have done.

Not everyone qualified as a journal keeper. In fact, a lot didn't. To keep the diet healthy, I screened out the juice fasters, crash dieters, extreme gourmets, and nutritional oddballs. I only wanted people without food issues who liked to eat but who also weren't closet superchefs or superchef groupies. I asked my volunteers to be 100 percent honest, and to help ensure it, I promised confidentiality.

Initially, I reached out to fifty women—friends and acquaintances who passed my "I am a regular eater" test. These were not people with a specific body mass index or weight-to-height ratio or any other quantitative measure of healthfulness. They just looked good to me. All of them said yes, they'd be happy to keep a diet journal. No problem.

I was off to a good start. Or so I thought. It turns out that even seemingly normal, well-adjusted women often have food issues. Only fourteen of the fifty women actually ponied up their diaries, even after heavy lobbying and some pleading on my part. The rest "lost" the journals, couldn't bring themselves to write down what they ate, or worried about being exposed as midnight nibblers. Eventually I enlisted another ten subjects, and I decided to keep a diary myself. That put my total number of journals at twenty-five. It was a small sample, but enough of one that I thought I had a good window on the eating habits of my target physical type.

Once I had the journals in hand, I began my data mining. I made a series of three-foot-long spreadsheets tracking my log keepers' breakfasts, lunches, dinners, and snacks. I tabulated calories, and I noted the numbers of skipped meals and repeated items. I jotted down bagel recurrences and the use of real butter versus butter spreads. I looked for favourite fruits and meals of choice. It was fascinating. Although no two women had the same exact daily calorie counts, each kept within her own 200ish-point spread. (In other words, if the journal keeper's normal tally was in the 1,600 range, she rarely exceeded 1,700 calories or fell under 1,500. So I found a remarkable degree of consistency, and no binge eating at all.)

Starbucks played such a big role in so many diets that I considered contacting CEO Howard Schultz for some sort of sponsorship. Manhattan women, I discovered, love hummus—more than anything. They're not above substituting a hunk of chocolate cake for a meal. And they don't eat all that much sushi, at least not in the week I tracked.

As the patterns of the diet began to come together, I decided to make some executive decisions. I would nix behaviours I didn't like, even if they were popular with my log keepers. For example, you won't find any references in the twenty-eight-day diet to skimmed milk, fake butter, or Splenda. You can't convince me that these low-fat or fat-free options are better tasting, more satisfying, and healthier than the Real Thing and the Whole Thing, in reasonable quantities. I try to stick with the least-processed possible options.

Some other things you won't see in the Manhattan Diet: snacking very late at night; skipping meals; eating half of your day's calories at dinnertime; consuming energy bars, diet fizzy drinks, or diet anything. All of these were popular with my dieters. You, of course, can substitute what you like. I'm just not going to suggest it, because that's not my recommendation for Manhattan Dieters.

The deeper I got into my journals, the more I knew I was on the right track. These women liked to eat, and they ate. I never got the sense of deprivation or hunger. When there was an episode of excess ("Quantities unknown, but a lot of food" read one description of a Chinese dinner), it was followed by an extra-long morning yoga session or a day of pared-back eating. In one case, when the dieter over-ate, she simply noted "out of town," too embarrassed to admit her transgression. (In person, she confessed that "out of town" involved a lot of Oreos.) Then she picked up where she left off, with heaped plates of beans, veggies, and brown rice. Instead of punishing herself for overeating, she just put the bad day behind her and moved on.

I felt like Santa on the lookout for the good and the naughty. I learned who had a weakness for coffee-cake mixture, who found solace in Greek yogurt, who loved to apartment-clean, and who made time for weekday breakfasts with her husband (even though she had already eaten once). I also began to identify patterns.

. . . .

How Do You Know You're Hungry?

Hunger is not the longing for a spoonful of Nutella, chased by another spoonful of Nutella. That's a craving. It's okay to satisfy a craving, but know when to stop. If you're truly hungry, your throat and mouth will be more sensitive. You'll feel a gnawing in the pit of your stomach, and you might feel a little nauseous. Don't let yourself get hungry. It's a recipe for all hell breaking loose. Here is a nutritionist's hunger scale, designed to help you measure how hungry you really are. The goal is to stay between 3 and 7, and the best way to do that is to eat something every three to four hours.

1. Insatiably hungry
2. Seriously hungry
3. Stomach-growling hungry
4. Slightly hungry
5. No longer hungry but not yet satisfied
6. Comfortably satisfied
7. Starting to feel full
8. Feeling quite full
9. Starting to get a stomachache from so much food
10. In actual pain from overeating

. . . .

The first thing I noticed was that the Manhattan Diet didn't cleave to any particular conventional diet wisdom. My journal keepers were catholic in their tastes. They liked M&M's, spaghetti, bacon, salami, low-fat yogurt, bagels, English muffins, chocolate chip cookies, cholesterol-lowering buttery spread, steak, Häagen-Dazs ice cream, french fries, Thai food, Italian food—pretty much all food. They weren't carb parsers or insane fat avoiders. Two-fifths of them often ate half or more of their calories at dinner time. One-fifth skipped breakfast, one-third skipped lunch, and one-third skipped dinner. One thing they didn't skip: dessert. Of my twenty-five subjects, twenty noted that they had dessert after dinner several times a week. They tended towards whole foods, but also they used Splenda, fat-free single cream, skimmed milk, and protein bars.

So here are the thirteen rules of the Manhattan Diet:

1. Eat what appeals to you.

2. Eat only when you're hungry.

3. Don't eat too much of whatever it is you're eating. My dia-rists' entries typically ran in small and specific increments: 40g chicken breast, .1 square chocolate, 90 ml red wine, 130g bean and sausage concoction, 80g mango, ½ tablespoon of low-fat grated Monterey Jack cheese; "½ of a 3-inch by 4-inch piece of chocolate mousse pie (all I felt like eating; I would have eaten more if I'd wanted to)" was not an atypi-cal dessert entry. Here's a typical dinner description: "4 yam fries, 3 tablespoons baba ghanoush, 5 small pieces bread, 3 baby carrots, 3 tablespoons Brie, 1 cracker, 90g rice, 60g meat substitute, 50g sautéed kale, 80g beetroot salad."

The good news is that the precision of their measure-ments reflected portion-control awareness, which is key for weight management. The bad news is that it drove me insane when I was tallying up calories: 25 calories here, 14 there. I longed for entries like "8-ounce steak with small baked potato, no butter, and 75g steamed broccoli." No such luck. In fact, there was no such entry or anything close to it. Dinners were more along the lines of this recipe by Italian cook Marcella Hazan: "2 chicken thighs sautéed with butter, lemon, rosemary, garlic, and wine; 75g orzo; 2 big helpings salad with olive oil and balsamic vinegar." Salmon steaks averaged 75–100g; pasta in the 100–175g serving; chicken was always under 175g.

Grazing in this borough has clearly replaced the tra-ditional breakfast, lunch, and dinner construction. Even restaurant menus reflect this trend. Only two of the twenty-five journal keepers ate anything like three distinct meals a day. Some women's logs reminded me of a baby's nursing schedule. Their entries couldn't even be broken into meals. They were just daylong feeds, with a new snack getting registered every half hour or so: 4 almonds, 3 forkfuls baked blueberry farmer cheese, 3 spelt pretzels, 1 small apple, 8 blue corn tortilla chips. This phenomenon leads me to rule number four (which is closely related to number two).

4. Don't let yourself go hungry. Travel with snacks. Stock up your desk with energy bars, almonds, cheese cubes, crackers, raisins, and dried fruit such as cranberries. Carry whatever you can reasonably and sanitarily cram into your handbag. In Manhattan, it's all about maintaining the blood-sugar level, which is why the days are structured as a series of small meals and snacks. (One caveat: there are people who can't stop at a small snack. If you're one of them, if one mini Snickers leads to a bagful, you'll probably want to consolidate the mini-meals I describe into three more traditional feedings. Just try not to go more than four hours without eating something.) What I call lunchfast—eating lunch or dinner foods at breakfast—was another big theme, which I associate with rule number one and the next rule.

5. Eat what your body craves. Just because it's 8 a.m. doesn't mean you have to have eggs, fruit, porridge, or Pop-Tarts. At midnight, how about a bowl of granola? That was actress Christine Baranski's default snack. Or why not some brown rice with minced beef and peas at 7:30 a.m., à la my friend Renee, a nurse? Myriam, a teacher, served herself a salad of lettuce, tomatoes, onions, and sardines at 10 a.m. almost every day. Mara's breakfast sounds like dinner at a yoga retreat: a mélange of beans, steamed Brussels sprouts, and quinoa salad, or roasted potatoes and beetroot along with sautéed Swiss chard. She's radiant and strong. You can see it

in how she carries herself, in her skin and her muscle tone. If nothing else, dinner at breakfast is an efficient way to use leftovers. It can be more filling and hearty than a bowl of cereal, and you won't be as hungry late in the day. Really, who needs conformity? When it comes to eating, Manhattan women don't worry about that. They're too busy.

6. Make habit your friend. Again and again I came across notes like "I don't mind eating the same thing a couple of days in a row" in reference to a tuna melt that did double lunch duty on Monday and Tuesday. Or "this porridge is the cornerstone of my diet. I eat it almost every morning." Novelist Lauren Lipton wrote that in keeping the diary, she realized she eats the same fifty things over and over again. That's plenty of variety and the basis of rule number seven.

7. Keep it simple. In fact, too much variety is actually a bad thing, because it can lead to overeating (think of how much you eat at a buffet, where there is incredible variety compared to when you order from a limited à la carte menu. More choices means more temptation to taste more).

When I read most diet books' twenty-eight-day eating plans, I'm often overwhelmed by the choices. They are meant to be motivational, I think, so that your diet doesn't feel mundane or repetitive. But as a busy person, I don't have the mental bandwidth or the refrigerator space to produce a sesame-sprouted wholemeal bread sandwich with 50 grams of fresh-roasted turkey, black olive tapenade, romaine lettuce, and onion for Monday's lunch; then chicken wraps with ginger marinade, grated carrots, and hummus on Tuesday; and some other completely different meal for every other lunch of the week. I'm a mom! I'm a professional! I'm busy! I say, poach a chicken or buy it roasted and serve it with different vegetables or make different salads or wraps.

Throw caution to the wind and eat the same thing a few days in a row. If you like spice-marinated salmon, why not make a double portion and have leftovers the next night? I often prepare the same dinner every night for weeks on end until I tire of it. For me, it's not so much about saving time—though that's an added plus—it's knowing what I like and sticking to it. If chicken Caesar salad every night is too monotonous for you, go with variety. It's easy to streamline my twenty-eight-day plan—just rejig things and keep the general calorie count in the same ballpark as the meal being replaced.

I have an innate suspicion of most packaged foods. I'm a decent cook, so I personally don't buy many, and I encourage you to cook from scratch. But I realize not everyone has the time or the inclination, and not all store-bought products are awful. Just be sure to look at the ingredients list so you know what you're getting. You can also mix and match some items you make yourself with a store-bought item or two. (For example, make a turkey filling from scratch but buy the taco shells and guacamole.)

My journal keepers were particularly fond of speciality grocery store Trader Joe's products, like chicken gyoza potstickers and spanakopita. Amy's Kitchen, a line of natural and organic prepared foods, was also mentioned repeatedly (especially her breakfast burritos). There are dozens of companies that produce partly assembled meals that are fresh and easy to put together. The online grocer Fresh Direct, Whole Foods, Trader Joe's, and many others offer stir-fry kits, premade shish kebabs, soups in a box, and all manner of products that make dinner preparation easier.

In this age of carbohydrate demonization, perhaps the biggest surprise to me was the popularity of pasta, rice, and bread products among my journal keepers. I'm not sure who is following those low-carbohydrate regimens, but my women are not. More than half had a bread product at breakfast, lunch, and dinner. One-third snacked on a bread item between meals. Pasta or rice was the single most popular dinner component. Only one diarist even approached a low-carb diet, and I know her to be a recent convert to the Paleo Diet, where you eat only the general types of foods that our hunter-gatherer ancestors would have eaten. Minced meat, yes; taco shells, no. Fish, yes; rice, no. Alligator, yes; cheese, no. Nevertheless, this diarist did allow herself multiple red velvet cupcakes during her week and even an occasional handful of toasted marshmallow jelly beans. That makes rule eight a no-brainer.

8. Love the grains: quinoa, spelt, Kamut (a type of wheat), rye. Make them whole and eat plenty of them.

9. Eat your veggies! Perhaps more predictably, the Manhattan Dieter's biggest friend was the salad, which dovetailed nicely with the "keep it simple" rule. Throw leftovers on a bed of greens, and you've got a meal. Salad was the most popular lunch item (nineteen of the twenty-five chose it at least once during the week), and at dinnertime it was second only to pasta or rice as the main event. If the journal keeper wasn't having salad as a main course, she had a small one on the side—and not necessarily a green salad. In some cases it was grapefruit and avocado; tomatoes, cucumber, and feta or goat's cheese; or tomatoes and olives. Salads, in fact, seemed to be the substitute of choice for an actual cooked vegetable. Five women skipped vegetables altogether at dinner at least once a week; only six women ate three or more vegetables with their dinner, and two of those were vegetarians.

A salad is a great backup, but it's not the same as a side of broccoli, roasted kale, or ginger carrots. And beware of salad dressing, because a few hundred calories can nestle comfortably in a few spoonfuls. The universal choice with my women was oil and vinegar, which is the hands-down healthiest way to give some spark to your leafy greens. Buy the absolutely best olive oil you can afford and use it sparingly—either with vinegar alone or in an easy vinaigrette. (In chapter 11, I have a vinaigrette recipe that is heavy on vinegar and mustard and light on oil.) I would avoid bottled fat free dressings for a variety of reasons, including the fact that you need oil to transport the vitamins in your salad greens to your blood.

The next rule almost goes without saying, but I will say it anyway because it doesn't seem to sink in, ever.

10. Avoid fast food. That means McDonald's, Dunkin' Donuts, KFC, and any other chain that serves ready-made meals. Manhattan Dieters avoid these places completely. Their pizza was artisanal (with broccoli and smoked sausage), and their burgers, served with toppings like bacon jam, were, too. If you don't count a Starbucks skinny latte or a Pret a Manger sandwich as fast food, the only reported instance among my journal keepers was a single dinner at International House of Pancakes. This woman polished off a stack of five buttermilk pancakes with a scoop of butter and a large helping of syrup, a scrambled egg substitute (go figure), four pieces of bacon, and coffee with single cream. Her total calories for the meal were about 1,600, which in itself explains the need for the no fast-food rule. Not every quick-serve meal is so calorie dense, but why go there?

11. Exercise. Just do it. My volunteers are pretty conscientious in this area. A few do something every day: take a yoga class, go to the gym, go for a run, ride a bike. Most mentioned exercise two or three times a week and any walking they did. I didn't ask for anyone to wear a pedometer, but estimating the distances they described and knowing what I myself do in the course of a day, I'd say the typical woman is walking between two and three miles a day. It's

been pretty well established that exercise doesn't make you lose weight and that the calories you burn during a workout amount to a couple of Snickers Minis. One basic rule I heard was that you burn 100 calories for every mile you walk or run. So while exercising is crucial to good health and healthy weight maintenance, it's not going to make you skinny. Only eating properly (and probably less) will do that.

12. By "eating properly," I don't mean just grilled fish and steamed spinach. I mean a balanced diet that both keeps you in line and allows you to cheat. It's okay to eat sweets. Put aside bananas and apples and other fruit (they came in third) that you know you should choose to satisfy a sweet craving. Instead, embrace your sweet tooth, as my journal-keepers did.

Twenty of them reported following dinner with dessert, whether a slice of cake, some cookies, or ice cream. That's more, by the way, than the number of women who recorded fish as a main course during the week and way more than those who chose steak, poultry, or eggs as a main dinner dish. About half had dessert at lunch time, and candy and cookies were the number one and two most popular. As for you, just don't overdo or underdo. The same applies to alcohol and rule number thirteen.

13. Bottoms up! This, I know, is a dicey one, because from a calorie-counting point of view, alcohol is kind of pointless. Red wine might boost your heart health with antioxidants and polyphenols, but nutritionally, it can't hold a candle to 200 grams of roasted butternut squash, sautéed kale, or a tomato salad. As one who's been there, I know alcohol also does bad things to willpower. But psychologically and emotionally, a glass of wine is sometimes what you want at the end of the day.

More than half my journal keepers reported having wine before, during, or after dinner (there were only five beer drinkers in the group and only three hard-liquor gals). If a glass of white or red or bubbly (which is lower in calories than "still" wine, by the way) is what you want, go for it, but don't drink more than 150 millilitres a day (or 350 millilitres of beer or 50 millilitres of hard liquor). And even though I often include a white wine spritzer or a glass of wine with dinner, you, of course, don't have to drink anything alcoholic at all. If you don't drink, don't start now!

The word *diet* can mean one of two things: the usual food and drink we consume every day or the restrictive intake of food we suffer in order to lose weight. The Manhattan Diet falls into the first class; it is what women here eat day in and day out. I want to go back to a point I made in chapter 2. Although it was unstated in the diaries, the mindfulness of the eating is clear. Manhattan women are strategic about what they eat. They are conscientious. There is very little impulse eating, with the exception of a handful of Cheerios snagged while pouring breakfast for a child or some Doritos from that same child's leftover lunch on the way to soccer practice.

That hyperawareness, more than anything else, informs the Manhattan Diet. Without counting calories, all of the women managed instinctively to stay within a specific calorie arc. It is the "be sensible" diet, the "no magic bullet" diet, the "no secret formula" diet. Just eat well, don't deprive yourself, don't go to bed full, and don't wake up famished. Even when you're not in Manhattan, you can do as the Manhattanites do. Most of the twenty-eight-day Manhattan Diet plan comes directly from my journal keepers. These are real, or variations on, meals my journal keepers have prepared, ordered at restaurants, or dialled in to eat at home.

When I finished putting together the twenty-eight-day regimen, I turned to Kim Diamond, a nutritionist and trainer whom I interviewed for chapter 9. I asked Kim to review the meals to make sure they were balanced and met accepted nutritional standards. Her main suggestions were to watch out for sodium, so go very easy on the salt as well as the bad, saturated fats (I got rid of a lot of cheese and trimmed back salty treats like olives and pretzels).

Because it is hard to get folic acid and a few other nutrients from food, Kim also suggested a daily vitamin. Finally, she thought I should remove wine from the menus. Although I understand her reasons—breast health and alcohol abuse, among others—I decided to keep it in because wine played such a big part in my dieters' journals. The meals are just suggestions, after all. As I mentioned in rule number 13, you don't *have* to drink wine. If you do, be sure to keep it to just 150 millilitres, and don't drink it every day. If you skip it on a day that I've included a glass, treat yourself some other way.

This gets to the bottom of the Manhattan Diet: it's flexible, if nothing else. It is both a blueprint and a concept. Take these ideas and run with them. Since the majority of my women kept their calories between 1,500 and 2,000, that was one guideline I used. You may have to adapt the portions for your size and activity level. I have often divided lunch into two minimeals, a favourite tactic of my diarists. Since twenty-one of twenty-five journal keepers included rice or pasta in their dinners, so do I.

Almost every diarist had the same daily breakfast and often repeated the same lunches and dinners a few days in a row. I am giving you many more options. You can find a handful you like and rotate them, or you can pick your favourite and have that every day. To that end, I include calorie estimates for each meal and snack, so if you want to substitute one for another, you can coordinate.

As a practical matter, if I suggest a chicken dinner one night, I tried to make lunch the next day chicken salad. That way, you're not stuck with an overwhelming number of leftovers. Any food that appeared repeatedly in my dieters' journals will be found in the diet, from wine to bread to pasta to candy. I also added in some of my favourite things to round out my dieters' choices, a few suggestions from experts, and a handful of recipes passed on to me by Cesare. Make sure to get your eight glasses of water a day, have fun, and as Cesare would say, *buon appetito*.

An asterisk after a dish indicates that a recipe for it is provided in chapter 11.

WEEK ONE

Jump-start your day Manhattan-style with a cup of coffee or tea. Use up to 2 teaspoons sugar or honey and 2 tablespoons whole milk. Or drink it black.
Calories: 70

DAY ONE
Approximate calories: 1,660
　　1 cup coffee or tea
　　Calories: 70

Breakfast
170g pot Greek yogurt, which is super-creamy, filling, and
　　high in protein. Top with 25g high-fibre granola.
Calories: 400

Morning Snack
1 clementine
Calories: 35

First Lunch
Chickpea salad: 100g chickpeas, diced tomato, chopped red
　　onion, flat leaf parsley, 1 teaspoon olive oil, and 2 teaspoons
　　red wine vinegar
Calories: 240

Second Lunch
½ turkey sandwich: 1 slice wholemeal bread, 50g fresh
roasted turkey, tomato, and mustard
Calories: 185

Afternoon Snack
1 chocolate-covered pretzel
Calories: 90

Cocktail
10 toasted almonds
1 white wine spritzer: 60ml white wine, 125ml soda water,
ice, and 1 slice lime or lemon
Calories: 110

Dinner
2 turkey tacos* with chopped tomato and chopped lettuce
1 corn on the cob
1 x 90ml glass white wine
Calories: 490

Evening Snack
1 square dark chocolate
1 cup herbal tea
Calories: 40

DAY TWO
Approximate calories: 1,650
1 cup coffee or tea
Calories: 70

Breakfast
1 fried egg
2 rashers bacon
1 slice wholemeal toast
2 clementines
Calories: 360

Morning Snack
1 apple
Calories: 110

First Lunch
Barley salad: 80g cooked barley, 2 tablespoons roasted corn
    kernels, 1 tablespoon finely chopped red pepper, 2 teaspoons
    sliced spring onion, 1 teaspoon olive oil, and 1 teaspoon red
    wine vinegar
Calories: 200

Second Lunch
2 turkey wraps: 50g roasted turkey, 1 tablespoon olive tap-
    enade, 4 slices tomato, two romaine lettuce leaves. Spread
    half of the tapenade on each lettuce leaf, layer on half of the
    turkey and two slices of tomato. Roll up and secure with a
    toothpick.
Calories: 160

Afternoon Snack
2 chocolate chip cookies
1 cup green tea
Calories: 130

Cocktail
2 Carr's Table Water crackers
25g mozzarella cheese
1 white wine spritzer: 60ml white wine, 125m soda water, ice,
    and 1 slice lime or lemon
Calories: 170

Dinner
125g pasta with 50g tomato sauce, 25g turkey mince, and
    1 tablespoon freshly grated parmesan cheese
100g sautéed broccoli
1 x 90ml glass wine
Calories: 415

Evening Snack
1 plum
Calories: 35

DAY THREE
Approximate calories: 1,670
1 cup coffee or tea
Calories: 70

Breakfast
1 serving lemony hummus* with 25 two-inch carrot sticks
(Hummus was a popular breakfast with my diary keepers, especially those who exercised a lot.)
Calories: 425

Morning Snack
50g dried apricots
Calories: 100

Lunch
1 organic Indian somosa wrap
125g pot natural full-fat yogurt with 2 teaspoons jam
Calories: 380

Afternoon Snack
1 banana
Calories: 100

Cocktail
10 mixed olives
1 glass soda water with lime
Calories: 50

Dinner
100g roasted chicken breast, skin removed
100g mixed salad leaves with 2 teaspoons vinaigrette*

100g quinoa
225g roasted broccoli
150ml glass wine
Calories: 545

Evening Snack
1 cup herbal tea

DAY FOUR
Approximate calories: 1,660
1 cup coffee or tea
Calories: 70

Breakfast
1 open panini: 1 slice wholemeal bread, scrambled eggs made with 3 whites and 1 yolk, 25g mozzarella cheese, 40g chopped lean roasted ham, and 1 teaspoon rapeseed oil
½ banana
Calories: 440

Morning Snack
½ banana
Calories: 50

First Lunch
1 serving butternut squash soup*
Handful of low-fat croutons
Calories: 110

Second Lunch
1 serving chicken salad*
100g mixed salad leaves with 2 teaspoons vinaigrette*
2 Carr's Table Water crackers
Calories: 300

Afternoon Snack
Let yourself be a little naughty. Have 25g Frosted Mini-Wheats
   or some other cereal.
Calories: 90

Dinner
1 serving red wine risotto*
1 serving sautéed broccoli*
Calories: 480

Evening Snack
2 biscuits
1 cup herbal tea
Calories: 120

DAY FIVE
Approximate calories: 1,700
   1 cup coffee or tea
   Calories: 70

Breakfast
1 serving Lauren Lipton's porridge* (Lauren attributes her tiny
   waistline to this dish, which she says is packed with fibre,
   calcium, and all kinds of other good stuff. It also keeps her
   going for hours.)
Calories: 575

Lunch
1 Greek salad pitta*
60g baba ghanoush
Calories: 422

Afternoon Snack
1 chocolate marshmallow tea cake
1 cup herbal tea
Calories: 110

Cocktail
25g lean roasted ham
225g pear slices
1 glass soda water with lime
Calories: 140

Dinner
1 serving shepherd's pie*
100g mixed salad leaves with 2 teaspoons vinaigrette*
1 x 125ml glass wine
Calories: 330

Evening Snack
2 squares dark chocolate with almonds
1 cup mint tea
Calories: 50

DAY SIX
Approximate calories: 1,650
1 cup coffee or tea
Calories: 70

Breakfast
½ wholemeal bagel with 1 tablespoon cream cheese
225g pear slices
Calories: 280

Morning Snack
4 asparagus spears wrapped in 50g lean roasted ham
Calories: 100

Lunch
Chef's salad: 150g mixed salad leaves, 50g roasted turkey breast, 50g lean roasted ham, 1 hard-boiled egg, 1 rasher bacon, and 1 tablespoon vinaigrette*
1 wholemeal roll
Calories: 490

Afternoon Snack
60g hummus with 5 two-inch carrot sticks
Calories: 130

Dinner
4-ounce steak
275g asparagus, drizzled with 2 teaspoons butter and 1 teaspoon freshly squeezed lemon juice
1 corn on the cob
1 x 125ml glass wine
Calories: 500

Evening Snack
3 Rolos or similar small chocolates
1 cup herbal tea
Calories: 80

DAY SEVEN
Approximate calories: 1,565
1 cup coffee or tea
Calories: 70

Breakfast
50g Cheerios or other oat cereal
125ml whole milk
1 banana
Calories: 340

First Lunch
100g mixed salad leaves with 2 teaspoons vinaigrette*
Calories: 50

Second Lunch
1 serving cooked pasta with 50g sautéed broccoli* and 1 tablespoon parmesan cheese
Calories: 315

Afternoon Snack
20 M&M's
Calories: 90

Cocktail
Mini-antipasto: 2 artichoke hearts, 3 olives, and 15g mozzarella *or* 15g dry pork salami
1 glass soda water with lime or lemon
Calories: 100

Dinner
1 serving prawns and beans* on Little Gem lettuce
1 wholemeal dinner roll
1 x 150ml glass wine
Calories: 480

Evening Snack
2 dried figs
Calories: 100

WEEK TWO

Jump-start your day Manhattan-style with a cup of coffee or tea. Use up to 2 teaspoons sugar or honey and 2 tablespoons whole milk. Or drink it black.
Calories: 70

DAY EIGHT
Approximate calories: 1,650
1 cup coffee or tea
Calories: 70

Breakfast
1 small oat scone
150g diced cantaloupe
125ml yogurt
Calories: 390

Morning Snack
12 green grapes
Calories: 60

First Lunch
1 serving spinach dip* with 10 two-inch carrot sticks
Calories: 150

Second Lunch
Tuna melt: 1 slice wholemeal bread, 75g tuna packed in oil
    and drained, a little mayonnaise, and 25g cheddar cheese
Calories: 350

Afternoon Snack
1 small apple
Calories: 85

Cocktail
1 slice tomato bruschetta*
1 white wine spritzer: 60ml white wine, 125ml soda water,
    ice, and 1 slice lime or lemon
Calories: 165

Dinner
1 serving sautéed spinach*
1 serving turkey chilli*
Calories: 330

Evening Snack
5 Gummy Bears
1 cup herbal tea
Calories: 45

DAY NINE
Approximate calories: 1,525
    1 cup coffee or tea
    Calories: 70

Breakfast
2 crispbreads with 2 tablespoons peanut butter and 2 teaspoons honey
Calories: 300

Morning Snack
300g diced cantaloupe
Calories: 120

First Lunch
1 serving tomato-watermelon salad*
Calories: 150

Second Lunch
1 tuna burger on rocket: 120g fresh-ground tuna, 1 teaspoon
   capers, 1 teaspoon red onion, and 1 teaspoon Dijon mustard, mixed into a patty and sautéed in a non-stick
   pan with olive oil spray
Calories: 190

Afternoon Snack
1 serving spinach dip* with 4 rice crackers
Calories: 140

Cocktail
150g sliced fennel with 1 teaspoon olive oil and salt to taste
1 white wine spritzer: 60ml white wine, 125ml soda water,
   ice, and 1 slice lime or lemon
Calories: 90

Dinner
200g butternut squash with 125g tomato sauce and 2 turkey
   meatballs*
1 steamed artichoke with 1 teaspoon olive oil and salt to taste
1 x 90ml glass wine
Calories: 345

Evening Snack
50g raisins
Calories: 120

DAY TEN
Approximate calories: 1,620
1 cup coffee or tea
Calories: 70

Breakfast
1 baked apple with raisins and 2 teaspoons cinnamon sugar
50g Greek yogurt
Calories: 290

Morning Snack
10 animal crackers
Calories: 100

First Lunch
1 Caesar salad*
Calories: 130

Second Lunch
1 turkey meatball* sandwich: 2 sliced meatballs on a small sub
   roll with 2 tablespoons tomato sauce
Calories: 300

Cocktail
5 radishes, 75g fennel, and 1 carrot sliced thin, with 1 teaspoon olive oil and salt to taste
1 glass soda water with lemon
Calories: 80

Dinner
125g roasted chicken breast*, skin removed
1 serving roasted root vegetables*
1 x 150ml glass wine
Calories: 500

Evening Snack
1 serving chocolate pudding* or chocolate peanut butter pudding*
Calories: 150

DAY ELEVEN
Approximate calories: 1,670
1 cup coffee or tea
Calories: 70

Breakfast
300g mixed blueberries and strawberries
170g pot Greek yogurt
2 teaspoons honey
Calories: 435

Morning Snack
3 digestive biscuits
1 cup tea
Calories: 50

First Lunch
1 serving roasted root vegetables*
Calories: 200

Second Lunch
1 chicken sandwich: 2 slices wholemeal bread, 75g chicken breast, 2 slices tomato, lettuce, and mustard
Calories: 340

Afternoon Snack
2 unsalted brown-rice cakes
Calories: 70

Dinner
1 serving chicken salad with radicchio and pine nuts*
1 slice wholemeal bread
Calories: 430

Evening Snack
50g fruit sorbet
Calories: 80

DAY TWELVE
Approximate calories: 1,600
1 cup coffee or tea
Calories: 70

Breakfast
1 spinach scramble*
1 slice wholemeal toast
Calories: 265

Morning Snack
1 Nakd bar
Calories: 100

First Lunch
100g steamed green beans with 1 tablespoon honey-Dijon
    dressing*
Calories: 80

Second Lunch
200g orzo pasta with spinach*
Calories: 317

Afternoon Snack
25g skinny popcorn
Calories: 125

Cocktail
25g vegetable crisps
1 glass soda water with lime
Calories: 130

Dinner
125g Tandoori salmon*

1 serving roasted radicchio*
80g cooked barley
1 x 150ml glass wine
Calories: 400

Evening Snack
½ pear poached in red wine
1 tablespoon Greek yogurt
Calories: 110

DAY THIRTEEN
Approximate calories: 1,560
1 cup coffee or tea
Calories: 70

Breakfast
250g cooked porridge with 2 teaspoons brown sugar and
    1 tablespoon raisins
1 banana
Calories: 290

Morning Snack
3 ginger biscuits
1 cup green tea
Calories: 100

Lunch
1 serving salmon salad*
100g mixed salad leaves with 2 teaspoons vinaigrette*
100g red pepper strips
1 wholemeal roll
Calories: 365

Afternoon Snack
6 cheese-flavoured Ritz crackers
Calories: 100

Dinner
1 serving pasta with black olives*
1 serving spring greens in spicy tomato sauce*
1 x 150ml glass wine
Calories: 550

Evening Snack
2 dates
1 walnut
Calories: 85

DAY FOURTEEN
Approximate calories: 1,630

1 cup coffee or tea
Calories: 70

Breakfast
40g puffed rice cereal with 150g blueberries, 6 almonds, and
    125ml whole milk
Calories: 290

Morning Snack
150g sliced mango
Calories: 110

First Lunch
200g minestrone soup
2 Ryvita crackers
Calories: 130

Second Lunch
½ roast beef sandwich: 1 slice wholemeal bread, 50g sliced
    roast beef, 1 slice tomato, and 2 teaspoons horseradish
    sauce
Calories: 180

Afternoon Snack
1 oat cookie*

1 cup tea
Calories: 90

Cocktail
1 serving roasted kale crisps*
1 glass soda water with lemon or lime
Calories: 100

Dinner
1 serving pasta with salmon and asparagus*
1 x 150ml glass wine
Calories: 435

Evening Snack
1 small slice apple pie
1 cup green tea
Calories: 225

WEEK THREE

Jump-start your day Manhattan-style with a cup of coffee or tea. Use up to 2 teaspoons sugar or honey and 2 tablespoons whole milk. Or drink it black.
Calories: 70

DAY FIFTEEN
Approximate calories: 1,600
1 cup coffee or tea
Calories: 70

Breakfast
2 oat and egg white pancakes*
150g blueberries
60ml Greek yogurt
Calories: 370

Morning Snack
4 dried-apple rings
Calories: 140

First Lunch
1 serving wholemeal linguine with roasted cauliflower*
Calories: 236

Second Lunch
100g Rocket salad: 50g rocket, 1 tablespoon feta cheese, 75g halved cherry tomatoes, 1 teaspoon oil, and 1 teaspoon vinegar
Calories: 85

Afternoon Snack
4 Ryvita
2 tablespoons edamame hummus
Calories: 100

Cocktail
12 cherry tomatoes, sliced, with 1 teaspoon olive oil and salt to taste
1 white wine spritzer: 60ml white wine, 125ml soda water, ice, and 1 slice lime or lemon
Calories: 140

Dinner
1 serving lentil soup*
100g quinoa
100g sautéed rocket
Calories: 340

Evening Snack
50g chocolate or fruit sorbet
Calories: 110

DAY SIXTEEN
Approximate calories: 1,620
Have an extra glass of water today.
1 cup coffee or tea
Calories: 70

Breakfast
¼ courgette frittata*
1 slice wholemeal toast
Calories: 310

Morning Snack
½ apple with 1 tablespoon farmer cheese, such as Neufchâtel
1 cup herbal tea
Calories: 75

First Lunch
100g mixed salad leaves with 2 teaspoons vinaigrette*
2 Ryvita crackers
Calories: 90

Second Lunch
1 serving lentil salad*
100g cooked brown rice
Calories: 325

Afternoon Snack
1 tablespoon chocolate chips
Calories: 70

Dinner
125g plaice fillet on parchment*
1 serving avocado and grapefruit salad*
100g wholewheat couscous
1 x 150ml glass wine
Calories: 590

Evening Snack
2 chocolate-dipped strawberries
Calories: 80

DAY SEVENTEEN
Approximate calories: 1,670
    1 cup coffee or tea
    Calories: 70

Breakfast
2 x 2½-inch buttermilk bran muffins
1 banana
Calories: 260

Morning Snack
1 orange
Calories: 100

First Lunch
1 serving avocado and grapefruit salad*
Calories: 240

Second Lunch
½ ham sandwich: 1 slice wholemeal bread, 50g roasted ham,
    15g mozzarella cheese, and mustard
Calories: 230

Afternoon Snack
25g pretzel chips
Calories: 100

Cocktail
100g thinly sliced cucumber in juice of ½ lime, chilli powder,
    and salt
1 white wine spritzer: 60ml white wine, 125ml soda water, ice,
    and 1 slice lime or lemon
Calories: 110

Dinner
2 prawn tortillas*
1 serving black bean, sweetcorn, and tomato salad*
Calories: 520

Evening Snack
1 Milky Way Mini
Calories: 38

DAY EIGHTEEN

Approximate calories: 1,630
   1 cup coffee or tea
   Calories: 70

Breakfast

1 tortilla filled with black bean, sweetcorn, and tomato salad*
1 tablespoon Greek yogurt
Calories: 270

Morning Snack

1 apple with 2 teaspoons peanut butter
Calories: 190

Lunch

1 spinach salad with artichokes*
1 slice wholemeal bread
Calories: 380

Cocktail

5 brown-rice cakes with 1 tablespoon olive tapenade*
1 glass soda water with lemon or lime
Calories: 90

Dinner

1 serving black-eyed beans with bacon and bitter greens*
100g cooked farro (a grain similar to barley; substitute barley
   if farro is unavailable)
1 x 150ml glass wine
Calories: 500

Evening Snack

1 Weight Watchers Chocolate Chip Brownie Bar
Calories: 130

DAY NINETEEN

Approximate calories: 1,500

1 cup coffee or tea
Calories: 70

Breakfast

1 fruit smoothie: 75g each pineapple, blueberries, and raspberries; 125g vanilla yogurt; and ice
Calories: 200

Morning Snack

1 mini bagel with 1 tablespoon cream cheese
Calories: 105

First Lunch

100g wholewheat couscous with 10 unsalted pistachio nuts
Calories: 130

Second Lunch

Romaine tuna wraps: 125g oil-packed tuna, 2 teaspoons mayonnaise, ½ shallot, 2 teaspoons chopped dill, plus 2 romaine leaves
1 wholemeal roll
Calories: 370

Cocktail

10 tortilla chips with 50g salsa
Calories: 100

Dinner

1 serving spinach dip* with 50g raw red pepper strips
1 Tesco Mexican Style Bean Burger
1 tortilla
Calories: 375

Evening Snack
1 serving chocolate pudding* or chocolate peanut butter
    pudding*
Calories: 150

DAY TWENTY
Approximate calories: 1,600
    1 cup coffee or tea
    Calories: 70

Breakfast
200g quinoa, with 60ml milk and 1 tablespoon brown sugar
150g blueberries
Calories: 340

First Lunch
1 serving bruschetta with beans*
Calories: 150

Second Lunch
1 serving chopped salad Niçoise*
Calories: 350

Afternoon Snack
1 serving carrot soup*
Calories: 100

Cocktail
75g boiled prawns with 2 tablespoons cocktail sauce
1 glass soda water with lime
Calories: 100

Dinner
200g roasted butternut squash cubes (see roasted root veg-
    etables*)
1 serving sautéed Swiss chard*

1 serving chicken Milanese*
Calories: 495

DAY TWENTY-ONE
Approximate calories: 1,665
1 cup coffee or tea
Calories: 70

Breakfast
1 spinach scramble*
½ wholemeal English muffin
Calories: 260

Morning Snack
50g snack mix: equal parts Cheerios, dried cranberries, and
  unsalted pistachios in the shell
Calories: 130

First Lunch
2 tablespoons hummus* with 6 two-inch carrot sticks
Calories: 75

Second Lunch
1 chicken Milanese* pitta: 1 wholemeal pitta, 50g chicken,
  1 tablespoon tapenade, 2 slices tomato, and 2 romaine
  leaves
Calories: 340

Cocktail
1 serving roasted kale crisps*
1 glass soda water with lime
Calories: 100

Dinner
1 serving tofu stir-fry*
100g cooked brown rice

1 x 150ml glass wine
Calories: 600

Evening Snack
3 Rolos or similar small chocolates
Calories: 90

WEEK FOUR

Jump-start your day Manhattan-style with a cup of coffee or tea.
Use up to 2 teaspoons sugar or honey and 2 tablespoons whole
milk. Or drink it black.
Calories: 70

DAY TWENTY-TWO
Approximate calories: 1,620
1 cup coffee or tea
Calories: 70

Breakfast
75g smoked salmon
1 tablespoon cream cheese
1 wholemeal English muffin
Calories: 310

Morning Snack
75g raw pumpkin seeds in the shell
Calories: 145

First Lunch
150g steamed broccoli with 1 tablespoon anchovy dip*
Calories: 120

Second Lunch
1 slice cheese pizza
Calories: 200

Afternoon Snack
1 nectarine
Calories: 110

Dinner
1 x 125g rosemary pork chop*
1 serving sautéed broccoli*
100g cooked brown rice
1 x 150ml glass wine
Calories: 570

Evening Snack
1 fruit ice pop
Calories: 80

DAY TWENTY-THREE
Approximate calories: 1,630
1 cup coffee or tea
Calories: 70

Breakfast
2 Kingsmill waffles
1 sliced banana
4 pecan halves
Calories: 330

Morning Snack
2 wholegrain rice cakes
Calories: 100

First Lunch
125g sugar snap peas
10 cherry tomatoes
Calories: 90

Second Lunch
1 egg salad sandwich: 2 slices wholemeal bread, 1 hard-boiled
    egg, 2 egg whites, 2 teaspoons mayonnaise, 1 teaspoon mus-
    tard, and a sprinkle of dill
Calories: 310

Afternoon Snack
1 lollipop
Calories: 60

Cocktail
20 peanuts
1 glass soda water with lime
Calories: 100

Dinner
125g roasted chicken*, skin removed
1 serving roasted radicchio*
175g sweet potato puree
1 x 150ml glass wine
Calories: 565

DAY TWENTY-FOUR
Approximate calories: 1,595
    1 cup coffee or tea
    Calories: 70

Breakfast
175g cottage cheese with 2 teaspoons honey
150g diced honeydew melon
Calories: 280

Morning Snack
2 kiwis
Calories: 100

First Lunch
25g prosciutto
1 dried fig
Calories: 125

Second Lunch
1 serving rocket and chestnut mushroom salad*
1 wholemeal roll
Calories: 300

Afternoon Snack
25g walnut halves (14 halves, or 7 walnuts)
Calories: 180

Cocktail
100g edamame beans
1 glass soda water with lime
Calories: 120

Dinner
1 serving wholewheat pasta with 100g sautéed spinach* and 1
    tablespoon parmesan cheese
Tomato salad: 1 tomato, 2 teaspoons finely chopped red onion,
    1 teaspoon olive oil and salt to taste
Calories: 350

Evening Snack
1 digestive biscuit
1 cup green tea
Calories: 70

DAY TWENTY-FIVE
Approximate calories: 1,675
    1 cup coffee or tea
    Calories: 70

Breakfast
1 small slice pumpkin bread
1 small nectarine, diced, mixed with 150g blackberries
Calories: 325

Morning Snack
3 lightly salted rice cakes
Calories: 75

First Lunch
1 serving mushroom soup*
2 Carr's Table Water crackers
Calories: 150

Second Lunch
1 toasted cheese sandwich with 25g cheese and 2 slices
   wholemeal bread, 1 rasher bacon, and 2 slices tomato
Calories: 325

Afternoon Snack
1 After Eight mint
Calories: 40

Cocktail
25g Kettle Lightly salted Chips
1 glass soda water with lime
Calories: 150

Dinner
150g rosemary-roasted trout*
1 serving asparagus salad*
1 slice wholemeal bread
1 x 150ml glass wine
Calories: 540

DAY TWENTY-SIX
Approximate calories: 1,740
   1 cup coffee or tea
Calories: 70

Breakfast
75g Swiss muesli with 125ml milk and ½ chopped apple
Calories: 420

Morning Snack
2 tablespoons dried cranberries with 1 tablespoon peanuts
Calories: 100

Lunch
100g loose leaf lettuce
1 serving Tuscan tuna salad*
2 x 4-inch bread sticks
Calories: 360

Afternoon Snack
2 wholegrain fig rolls
Calories: 110

Cocktail
25g vegetable crisps
Calories: 130

Dinner
1 serving mussels in sake*
200g cooked brown rice
25g green beans with Asian-style dressing*
1 white wine spritzer: 60ml white wine, 125ml soda, ice, and
   1 slice lime or lemon
Calories: 450

Evening Snack
30 green grapes
Calories: 100

DAY TWENTY-SEVEN
Approximate calories: 1,520
> 1 cup coffee or tea
> *Calories:* 70

Breakfast
1 wholemeal English muffin, 1 poached egg, 1 slice tomato, 125g lean roasted ham, and 15g grated cheddar cheese
Calories: 300

Morning Snack
1 pear
2 walnuts
Calories: 150

First Lunch
Heart of palm salad: 150g heart of palm, 175g tomato chunks, 100g Little Gem lettuce, 2 teaspoons olive oil, 2 teaspoons red wine vinegar, 1 teaspoon parsley, and salt and pepper to taste
Calories: 170

Second Lunch
50g sliced roasted turkey breast with mustard on 2 Ryvita crackers
Calories: 140

Cocktail
Seeds from one medium pomegranate with 25g Gorgonzola
1 white-wine spritzer: 60ml white wine, 125ml soda water, ice, and 1 slice lime or lemon
Calories: 210

Dinner
1 x 125g salmon burger
300g sautéed courgette and tomato
100g quinoa

1 x 90ml glass wine
Calories: 420

Evening Snack
2 strawberry-flavoured liquorice twists
1 cup fruit tea
Calories: 60

DAY TWENTY-EIGHT
Approximate calories: 1,630
1 cup coffee or tea
Calories: 70

Breakfast
2 x 4-inch buttermilk pancakes with 150g blueberries and
    1 tablespoon maple syrup
Calories: 310

Morning Snack
10 almonds
Calories: 70

First Lunch
225g curried cauliflower soup
Calories: 70

Second Lunch
100g mixed salad leaves, 25g peas, 100g wholewheat
    couscous, 2 tablespoons dried cranberries, 25g blue
    cheese, and 1½ tablespoons vinaigrette*
Calories: 330

Afternoon Snack
20 chocolate-covered raisins
Calories: 85

Cocktail
10 Warburtons Pitta Chips
Calories: 130

Dinner
25g rocket topped with 1 serving black bean, sweetcorn, and
    tomato salad*
125g grilled mahi-mahi (tilapia and monkfish are good alter-
    natives) marinated in lime and coriander
100g wholewheat couscous
1 x 125ml glass wine
Calories: 475

Evening Snack
1 oat cookie*
1 cup herbal tea
Calories: 90

7

White Truffle Risotto and Other Dilemmas

How We Order in Restaurants

In my experience, restaurants are not a dieter's friend. The food they serve is fatty. They trick you into overeating with clever lighting and atmosphere. Then they ply you with wine, which weakens your defences against bread, dessert, and cheese trays. In Manhattan you have to be doubly on guard, because there are so many more places trying to lure you in for a meal—about seven thousand, including nine of the country's top forty eateries. In terms of the number of restaurants per person, that easily beats San Francisco, which likes to claim the title of City with the Most Restaurants per Capita, and every other burg with dibs on the honour, too.

Upping the ante in Manhattan, if you have a pulse or social aspirations, you're expected to check out every flash-in-the-pan that opens to rave reviews, even as you maintain your *Vogue*-ish size 2 (UK size 6) figure. Walk into hot spots like Chef's Table at Brooklyn Fare, Ma Peche, or ABC Kitchen, and you'll see that the restaurants aren't only full, they are full of the skinniest, most chic people you've ever seen. They look like they spend most of their days detoxing on the Organic Avenue cleanse and in the gym but then show up tucked into a corner table brandishing a fork and a spoon. How is it possible?

I will tell you: they're not eating—not much, anyway. They're certainly not averaging the 1,000- to 1,500-calorie meals that restaurants are known for. In these places, 1,000 to 1,500 calories is chump change. As I write, I am studying the menu for the Breslin, created by Manhattan's chef crush of the moment, April Bloomfield. There are poussin fried in duck fat, peanuts fried in pork fat, and chips fried three times over, no fat identified. A diner could top 1,500 cals just in appetizers. But Manhattan women don't. Instead, they practise the art of dining while not eating.

Women here study a menu. They order. And then they push the food around on their plates. They split a main course with a friend, order two appetizers, or request the sauce on the side. They ask for no butter, no oil, or no dairy.

It drives waiters and chefs crazy. "It's like, 'Okay, I'm here, I made it. It's helping my status, my self-esteem, and I'm going to negate the reason I'm here and change the food,'" says Brian Buckley, a consultant who also teaches at the International Culinary Institute. "It's 'Look at me. I brought my own salad dressing. I'm running the show.' Ten to fifteen years ago, people didn't eat out to be healthy. They ate out to eat."

I have to cop a semi-guilty plea to this sort of behaviour. Given the choice, I am one of those sauce-on-the-side, prawn cocktail, sushi girls. Sometimes I wonder at the Freudian implications of the fact that I married Cesare when my eating life is so fraught with restrictions and guilt. Everyone thinks it's so fantastic to live with a chef, and there are many upsides, as I've detailed elsewhere (free-flowing Tuscan olive oil, organic broccoli, creamy imported cannellini beans).

But I am telling you, as a restaurant dining partner, Cesare is Kryptonite. We study a menu, and he doesn't just choose three courses. He orders from every category in multiples—anything that sounds even vaguely appealing. It's even worse when he knows the owners or the chefs, which is almost always, because they bring complimentary dishes. Instead of just having to taste what he picks, I also have to sample all of the dishes he didn't.

For example, the restaurant at the Four Seasons is one of my favourite eateries. Just stepping into the Grill Room makes me feel glittery and sleek. There are plenty of simple, sensible things on the menu. I like the Dover sole and the seafood platter, which is just a mound of delicious steamed lobster, crab, and prawns. But before I can ask for either, Julian, owner and friend of Cesare, sweeps in and produces white truffle risotto, foie gras, and quince and bottles of Barolo and Sassicaia wines.

Cesare won't let me not taste everything. So I do, using my fail-proof strategy: I nibble—barely. I will have half a bite of the duck and use my little finger to swipe up a drip or two of red wine sauce reduction. I use a teaspoon to scoop up a few grains of risotto. Occasionally, when it is something flash fried in salty, irresistibly crunchy, diet-defeating batter, I lapse and eat more than I was planning to. I just can't help myself.

But usually I don't cave. I taste everything but eat almost nothing. Sometimes we will get home from a dinner out and I will end up eating a handful of almonds or another snack because I am still hungry. It seems pointless to dine out this way, but if I didn't, I fear I'd be the size of the Chrysler building, just shorter and with no write-up in the American Institute of Architects' guide.

My paranoia isn't irrational. Nutritionists will list a dozen reasons why it's better to eat at home, from knowing what the ingredients are to portion control. Yet I'm not saying dieters should be housebound. Cesare would kill me. It's unrealistic, anyway, since the average American packs away about a fifth of her meals—and more than a third of her calories—in restaurants, according to the *Journal of the American Medical Association*. The restaurants could be Per Se, Charlie Trotter's, Osteria Mozza, or another temple of conscientious cookery where you can get your sea bream poached and your locally grown, organic baby spinach gently steamed. But more likely it's the Taco Bell, the golden arches, or some other fast-food joint, which are the destinations of 75 percent of U.S. eaters when they dine out.

The problem is that restaurants of any stripe are calorie minefields, even with new laws in some states requiring fast-food operators to post calorie counts. Most diners have no idea how many calories are in a Big Mac or a small side salad. In studies done in the last few decades, normal-weight eaters have consistently guessed wrong at calorie counts by about 20 percent, and the overweight fared worse. They falter by as much as 40 percent, with some thinking they eat half as many calories as they actually do.

The problem has to do with the size of the meal, says Brian Wansink, the Cornell professor I quoted earlier. The bigger the meal, the more likely it is that the eater will misdiagnose the number of calories. Given that the overweight tend to eat larger portions than their skinny counterparts, they're more likely to flub the count.

In one study I read, the more artery-clogging the food, the more mistaken the diners' counting was. For off-the-charts fattening dishes like fettuccine Alfredo and cheese fries, 99 percent got the calories wrong. Those cheese fries—which, by the way, came laced with ranch dressing—totalled 3,010 calories. But subjects put the dish in the 1,000-cal range. They also underestimated fat levels by

44 grams, saturated fat by 15 grams, and sodium content by 1,557 grams. When it came to healthier dishes like grilled chicken breast, the guesstimates were a little more accurate, but not impressively so. Some 73 percent of the subjects missed the calorie mark on those meals.

Perceptions apparently are swayed by the unlikeliest factors, including the size of the plate, the colour of the room, and where you sit in a restaurant. One new study revealed that even the order of the courses comes into play. In the experiment, diners were shown a piece of cheesecake and then a hamburger, then a fruit salad and a hamburger. When the subjects saw the cheesecake first, they estimated that the burger was just 780 calories. But when they saw the fruit salad first, they pegged the burger at 1,041 calories. (Conclusion: don't order fried mozzarella sticks as an appetizer.) Another research paper, published in the *Journal of Consumer Psychology*, showed that adding a salad to a meal prompted eaters to think they were eating fewer calories than they would have eaten without the salad.

I can totally sympathize with the tendency to get it wrong. Even trained experts can have trouble sizing up a restaurant dish's calories. What's interesting, of course, is that participants are more likely to undercount rather than overcount. Sociologists call it *optimistic bias*, or as I spell it, d-e-n-i-a-l. Optimistic bias is what happens when you're unreasonably sunny about a plan and its risks. Optimistic bias helped inflate the property bubble that burst in 2008. It also explains why newlyweds expect their marriage to last a lifetime and smokers think they're less likely than other smokers to get lung cancer. In a restaurant, optimistic bias is ordering a plate of french fries "for the table."

That's a trick I know well. And clearly, so do a lot of other ladies around town—you know, the no-cream-in-the-soup crowd, the no-butter-in-the-risotto customer, your garden-variety fat-phobe. Chefs, maître d's, and waiters tell me that these clients might say they want to eat light, but that's not how they actually order. When Cesare had a restaurant called Beppe, he made a point of including a poached fish and chopped salad on the menu, at my insistence. The items were so unpopular that he dropped them. His best sellers? Deep-fried chicken and deep-fried Tuscan fries, both of which came liberally sprinkled with delicious handfuls of deep-fried sage, rosemary, and thyme.

Tom Piscitello, the manager of A Voce, an upscale Italian place on Madison Avenue, says his female clientele come in after work with friends, and the first thing they do is order a green salad. But then they drink a couple of glasses of wine, and they start ordering dishes like cassoncini—a type of fried ravioli with a creamy cheese or fresh ricotta stuffing served with hunks of grilled bread drizzled with olive oil.

Brian Buckley, the restaurant consultant I quoted earlier, can go on for hours about this brand of diner. He comes back to the sauce-on-the-side conceit. Although his restaurateur clients are happy to serve main courses and side dishes that way, it's a pointless exercise, he says. Not only do diners dip their fingers into the sauce for multiple tastings, sometimes they are so enthusiastic, they end up wiping the bowl clean. When a woman is out to dinner with her husband or a date, she will order the spinach for herself and the hash browns for her companion. "The man will roll his eyes," Buckley says. "That means 'I won't be getting any of that.' And she will eat his hash browns and the spinach, too, because it's good for her."

It doesn't have to be this way. If you listen to Manhattan chefs and other foodies, restaurant customers could dispense with the games by simply eating better in everyday life. But the way many women eat out tends to mirror the way many Americans eat in general—that is, badly. Mireille Guiliano wrote about the problem in *French Women Don't Get Fat*, and it's a favourite theme with everyone from whole-foods hero Michael Pollan to author Harvey Levenstein. There is so much food in this country, the theory goes, that U.S. eaters are indifferent to it.

They "eat and run rather than dine and savour," writes Levenstein in his book *Revolution at the Table*. Quantity, not quality, is the measure of a good restaurant meal, a cultural bias that affects every diner's experience. If Americans enjoyed their food more, they wouldn't have to order sauce on the side or insist on skimmed milk or sole sautéed without butter. They could order their own hash browns and eat them, too.

I don't want to overstate the point, but because New York is physically closer to Europe than most of the rest of the United States, I think Manhattanites are nearer in lifestyle to the Continent's citizens. That's one of the reasons my circles of acquaintances are thinner than your typical American urbanites, and it's why more upscale restaurants here can get away with portions that would seem microscopic in the heartland. People here are even willing to pay *more* to eat *less* if they are getting quality ingredients and a big-name chef at the stove.

Mark Ladner oversees the kitchen at Del Posto. This restaurant is one of a dozen or so in the Mario Batali empire and is a destination for Wall Street deal makers, couples out on a special night, and gourmet tourists. In the autumn of 2010, Mark became the first chef in an Italian restaurant since 1974 to win a four-star review from the *New York Times*. Because he's using specialized items, like beef from grass-fed cows and handmade pasta, that are expensive for him to buy, Mark keeps the portions of his $95 (£60) five-course meal and his $125 (£80) seven-course meal pretty small. Order his beef rib eye with fried potatoes, Parmigiano-Reggiano, ruchetta and tomatoes, and the meat will tip the scale at seven ounces (200 grams). Spaghetti with Dungeness crab will arrive tableside at 100 grams. Compare that to the $27.95 (£17) steak Toscano at Olive Garden, which weighs in at twelve ounces (350 grams), or the chain's $15.25 (£10) serving of capellini pomodoro, which at 700 grams could serve seven Del Posto customers. Although Mark has barely heard a peep about portion size from his Manhattan clients, diners from other places can get cranky about it. "People complain, but it's one of those things," he says. "Mostly people who are complaining see value in volume. Manhattan diners have a better understanding and appreciation of quality. If you're getting high quality, you're not going to get a pound of it."

Eric Ripert, the chef at the four-star fish temple Le Bernardin, pins the disconnect between enjoyment of food and portion size on American culture. Eric grew up in Andorra, a thumbnail-sized country in the Pyrenees, wedged between France and Spain. People there eat what they need—sometimes a little more, sometimes a little less. And they have long lives to boot. There isn't the kind of obesity problem there is in the United States, and there isn't the accompanying hand-wringing. What Eric has observed about Americans is that they can't go two hours in a car without stocking up on food and drink, and then their reaction is to feel remorse about it.

Eric is mystified by reporters who ask him about his food guilt trip. "I have none! This is an American thing to have a guilt trip about what you eat. I regulate myself. I'm not obese or skinny. I'm just living the way I like to live. I have found my balance. I like indulgences on the weekend, but the day after, without forcing myself, I will eat light." He thinks Americans need to have a different approach to eating, not just in restaurants but in every aspect of feeding and nourishing. "The fact you are guilty when you put food in your mouth has consequences," he says.

At the same time, the chef sympathizes with Manhattan women's preoccupation with dieting. "It's ugly, but women are on the market. Men can be overweight, but they are hypocritical when it comes to women," Eric tells me. He describes a female friend, a beautiful former model who diets constantly, does juice fasts, and spends all day at the gym "running like a hamster." He grimaces and throws up his hands. "She has a terrible life."

Mark and Eric seem to be saying the same thing, in different ways: most Americans don't know how to eat or enjoy food. I wonder if this is the foodie secret and the explanation of why all the best and newest Manhattan restaurants are filled with the slenderest clientele possible. Are they all closet Europeans? Are we doomed

because we didn't grow up in Aix-en-Provence or some other for-
eign city where the citizens *dine and savour* rather than *eat and run*?

. . . .

Dining Out Tips from the Pros

If you're trying to decide between olive oil and butter for your
bread at a restaurant, go for the oil. You're likely to use more
oil on each piece of bread, but you will be satisfied quicker,
end up eating less bread, and consume fewer total calories.
That's, at least, what happened when Brian Wansink conducted a test on diners at an Italian restaurant. The customers who were given olive oil consumed 26 percent more fat
than those who got butter, but they ate 23 percent less bread.

A salad at lunchtime isn't always satisfying. Instead,
choose a sandwich, says celeb nutritionist Heather Bauer
(who, among her other accomplishments, helped supermodel
Tyra Banks go down three dress sizes). It is a controlled way to
have your carbohydrates, and you can pack in extra nutrients
by using spinach instead of lettuce as well as extra tomatoes.

Beware the brunch menu, says restaurant consultant
Brian Buckley. You think you're just ordering an omelette or
some French toast, but then, voilà, out comes the bacon,
maple syrup, corn bread, and other goodies—all of which can
be hard to resist (especially after the free Buck's Fizz).

Another restaurant trick is the dessert trolley, says Buckley.
Although many diners are able to resist a sweet at the end of
the meal if they are simply presented a menu, their willpower
evaporates if they come face-to-face with a tray displaying dense
chocolate cake, a decadent tiramisu, or other goodies.

Thinking about a night at a Mexican restaurant?
"That doesn't mean you're stuck with chicken tacos," says
Manhattan nutritionist Sharon Richter. Some other more
interesting choices include ceviche, any type of fajita (just

go easy on the tortillas, cheese, and sour cream), or tortilla soup, without the fried tortilla strips. Menus "don't always give people all the information," says Richter.

. . . .

I decide to check in with Dana Cowin, the longtime editor of *Food & Wine*. As part of her job, Dana eats at great, upcoming, established, reinvented, and every other sort of restaurant, day in and day out. We don't see each other often, but when I ask her to lunch to talk about restaurant meals, she is immediately game.

Dana has been svelte as long as I've known her, which is more than twenty years, even as she's feasted willy-nilly in her role as a foodie arbiter. She says the trick in restaurants is to order what you want but just sample it. Take the time to taste each spoonful. Learn something about food from your meal. We are lunching in a place called Aquavit, and I notice immediately that the menu is full of dieting booby traps. Many dishes come bathed in cream sauce. The Chatham cod is done in brown butter, the elk in a rich red wine sauce, and the french fries in truffle oil.

Dana skips those, settling quickly on a herring sampler and bowl of bouillabaisse. She explains her choices: the restaurant is Scandinavian and known for herring. The sampler offers something she might not get elsewhere and should showcase the restaurant's strength. It also promises to be light. Ditto for the bouillabaisse, a fish soup that isn't a Scandinavian speciality but that could shed light on the skills of a new chef, Marcus Jarnmark.

As we eat, I worry that Dana might think I'm a freak, but I can't help but study her mouth and how she chews. She doesn't just not gulp things down; she eats slowly and carefully. She is savouring! It's what Mark and Eric and the other foodies are talking about. Even when I am picking at something, I don't stop to really appreciate what's going into my mouth. At the end of our meal, a third of Dana's food is untouched, and yet she seems so satisfied.

I start to form a conclusion: Dana and Mark and Eric are in cahoots. It's the foodies' corollary of the mindful eating I described in chapter 2, in which women focus on every mouthful, counting each calorie and considering fat content, cholesterol, and carbs. Here the key is to be both mindful in the sense of watching what you eat and mindful in relishing every bite.

Yet there is something about this approach that keeps nagging at me. Let's be honest: foodies eat differently from the rest of us. Set aside for a moment the larger issue of the American culture of overkill—bucket o' cookies and the Luther burger, a cheeseburger served on a deep-fried doughnut. Say Americans had better diets in general. Say they appreciated good food more. I'm still not sure that this would translate to a universally more gratifying restaurant experience. That's because of another restaurant truth that no one has mentioned yet: chefs and their dieting diners don't trust one another; in fact, they're at war.

On one side, there are the customers: the ones who *say* they want to eat skinny, but really don't—the folks who drive chefs nuts. There are also some diners who really don't eat: the lettuce leaf-seeking, steamed white rice-loving, no butter and no oil crowd. They are a little easier to serve because they at least stick to their guns.

On the other side of the divide are the chefs. Their problem is that they revel in fat: the velvety-mouth feel, the flavour it adds, the satisfaction it delivers to the brain, the magic that it works in cooking—from the crispy crust on a perfectly cooked steak to the flakes in the pâte brisée.

Looking at the two camps, I see no common ground. There are the food avoiders on one side and the food providers on the other. As I said, war.

Yet the chef's job is to keep the restaurant running, to lure in the dieter and non-dieter alike, the healthy and the not so healthy. So what does he do? He plays games.

Last night, for example, I was out with some friends at a restaurant and ordered the Jonah crab salad with avocado, ceviche sorbet, and spiced popcorn crisp. It sounded delicious and calorie correct. Crab is high in cholesterol but only about 30 calories an ounce, ceviche is practically calorie-free, and avocado is packed with omega-6 fatty acids and fibre. I felt safe.

What the chef left out of the description, however, was the mayonnaise. And there was a lot of it. I can't believe this was an accident. The chef knows that most Manhattan diners are somewhat health-conscious. Include the word *mayonnaise* in an item description and chances are, orders will plummet. That explains the abundance of loaded, evocative terms on menus. You know the ones: *day-boat, free-range, organic*—any words that conjure up healthy critters in the wild. It also explains the mysterious lack of the naughty bits: terms like *butter, oil,* and *mayonnaise*.

"I wouldn't say menus are deceptive," says Buckley, the restaurant consultant. He chooses instead to call them "conveniently descriptive."

It's not that it would be so hard to give customers a helping hand. Butter, oil, and salt make everything taste better, but even chefs acknowledge that they could squeeze out a few calories without diners even noticing. When a research team from Pennsylvania State University surveyed more than four hundred chefs, almost all said they could cut the calorie content of their food by 10 to 25 percent without their customers knowing.

Instead, chefs persist with menu tricks to pass dishes off as healthier than they are. In describing desserts, they list the apricot compote before the gingerbread to create the impression that it's a fruit dessert with cake instead of the other way around. They promote the Trojan horse of menu items: the Caesar salad with grilled chicken. You might think this is a healthy choice. It certainly sounds like it, with its base of romaine lettuce and grilled bird. But thanks to the oil, cheese, and fried croutons piled on top, the calorie count in a typical main-course-sized Caesar is in the 2,500 range, says Buckley. In case you're counting, that's more calories than a Big Mac and fries combined or the Cheesecake Factory's chocolate tower truffle cake, a 1,670-calorie slab of saturated fat.

The list of misleading menu items is endless. There are bisques, which sound filling and good for you, but they're made with double cream. The tuna melt's major component is fish, but it's also loaded with mayo and cheese. There are the obvious red flags: anything with the words *deep-fried*, *pan-fried*, *basted*, *batter-dipped*, *breaded*, *creamy*, *crispy*, *scalloped*, *Alfredo*, *au gratin*, or *cream sauce*. Yet even the word *roasted* can signal trouble ahead. Roasting is healthy, right? Actually, says Buckley, it's restaurant code for drenched in butter. "The last step in any fish that is roasted is to spoon butter over it," he says. "Somehow that is never mentioned in the description."

What's a dieter to do? There are plenty of strategies for eating healthy and well that might not satisfy the foodie police, but at least they'll keep you out of Spanx body shapers. Some women I spoke to view restaurants in the larger context. They eat what they want when they are out to dinner but cut back the day before and the day after. Others eat only half of their order, forgo wine, or choose the two-appetizer route. One woman told me that she asks the waiter to bring the bread basket first as a test of willpower (this is a little masochistic, in my book), and another never drinks wine because it's a waste of calories. Quite a few use online menu sites to screen a restaurant before making a reservation.

There are those who have learned to dodge invitations from friends who pressure them to overorder, and there are those who eat in groups as a way of keeping their intake down. Donna Sexton, who gained more than one and a half stone when she moved to Manhattan from Australia, has slimmed back down by frequenting a rotisserie, Chirping Chicken, five days a week, taking home half a roasted chicken (dark meat only, which is more filling). She splurges at fancier places on the weekend.

Robin Reif, a marketing executive, narrows her choices. She sticks to fish and salad, with a few restaurant-specific exceptions. At Trattoria Dell'Arte, a popular Italian spot, she allows herself to get fried Jewish artichokes but asks for an extra napkin to "squish out the grease." If she's at an Indian restaurant, she'll order tandoori chicken, and when she's dining Chinese she'll order green beans and rice. "I ask for the beans extra well done with hardly any oil," she notes. "The oil on the green beans is enough to moisturize the rice. I eat with chopsticks, which helps [me] take smaller bites."

The most foolproof strategy I heard was to grill the waiter (not literally). Does *poached* mean in water? One friend of a friend neglected to ask this when she dined at Il Mulino, an elegant, old-style Italian restaurant in Greenwich Village. Poached turned out to be cooked in olive oil. "It's called *fried*," says the woman with disgust. "I ate around it. I know rationally that one time won't make a difference, but psychologically, I can't and won't do it. Why should I? As much as I know the chef wants to show off what he's created, I want to eat what I want to eat."

Manhattan Diet Secrets

- *Really enjoy what you eat, but just eat less of it.* This is the best dieting advice ever. The bonus: you can take the left-overs home for tomorrow's lunch.

- *If that's not the kind of advice you're looking for when you're at a restaurant, there are other tactics.* For one, the best offence is a good defence. Many Manhattan Dieters have fallback meals and even restaurant genres. Japanese is a no-brainer. At steak houses, the go-to menu item should be the raw bar: you can't go wrong with clams and oysters or even steamed prawns and lobster. And never underestimate a good roasted chicken.

- *Research is your friend.* Checking menus online before making a reservation can help you to settle on a meal ahead of time.

- *Don't believe what you read.* If you have doubts about what is in a dish or how flexible the chef will be in altering it, just ask the waiter, advises Manhattan nutritionist Sharon Richter. "I always say don't be afraid to ask. It's a service industry. It is their job to serve you." And don't worry, no question is too obvious, including "I'm about to go out drinking with my friends. What should I do beforehand?" Richter's suggestion: eat bananas, so that you're not drinking on an empty stomach.

- *If all else fails, hold your chef accountable.* April Bloomfield, the chef at the Breslin, is known for refusing to take any sort of special request from a customer. In a Menupages .com post that went viral, a diner named Erin complained that Bloomfield refused to cook her pregnant friend's steak medium well-done, refused to serve her salad with dressing on the side, and would not make scrambled eggs well-done. The story was picked up by the the *New York Post* and repeated elsewhere on food websites. Score one for the customer.

8

Okay, We Cheat

How We Break the Rules

It's 1:05 p.m. I am on the seventh floor of Bloomingdale's at 59th Street and Lexington Avenue. To be precise, I am threading my way through the bedding department, a beachhead of puffy duvets and flouncy throws for twins, queens, and kings. Generations of silkworms have given their lives in the service of the tassels on display. To my right is a model boudoir: sensuous, overstuffed, and beckoning. To my left are piles of cheery floral percales.

But like the other thirty-five women in line, I am not here for the Vera Wang Love Knots or the Ralph Lauren Jamaica Paisley. Nor am I considering the $150 (£90) Egyptian cotton bath towels or the matching combed-cotton bath mats. I have come for something more delicious than sheets with a seven-hundred thread count, something more irresistible than goose down and much better than plush terry.

It's lunchtime, and that means one thing: I am here for the frozen yogurt.

If New Yorkers have an Achilles's-heel snack, it is soft-serve frozen yogurt. Froyo, as it's called, is one of those faux diet foods, made with corn syrup, sodium, and white sugar but without the good-for-you active cultures that are in actual yogurt. Yet Manhattanites can't get enough of froyo. Their addiction has given birth to a not-so-small village of frozen yogurt shops: Pinkberry, Red Mango, Yorganic, Berrywild, and Eskamix are a few that come to mind. Today I'm at the granddaddy of them all, Forty Carrots, a luncheonette inside Bloomie's that has been dispensing twirls of plain, coffee, and other flavours to queues of shoppers since the Ford administration. Fans describe the yogurt's assets in italic superlatives. The *best* frozen yogurt, the *creamiest*, the *tastiest*.

I'm not an aficionado, so I can't vouch for the superiority of the Forty Carrots brand. However, I suspect that tastiness and creaminess aren't the main attractions. No, the headliner here would be the calorie count: about 350 for a really generous small serving—that's half the number in a bowl of Pret a Manger lentil soup or a tuna salad baguette. A large serving will tip the calorie counter at 450. Why go for a balanced meal when you can have a frozen yogurt the size of your head, with just a gram of fat per 25g? In line, I am standing behind a svelte fifty-something woman dressed in black from head to toe. She tells me she's been a daily customer for years because "it's fast and fun and the best lunch."

So, yes, in spite of their sanctimony and their sushi, edamame, and protein shakes, a great number of Manhattan women are not the healthiest of eaters. They might not mind washing Swiss chard three times, stripping off the leaves, chopping off the stems, and steaming it all before drizzling it with extra virgin olive oil and sea salt from Brittany. But not everybody does that. There are plenty of Manhattan dieters who cheat—and who cheat often.

They pay lip service to whole, unprocessed foods and locally grown veggies, then they stock their shopping trolleys with Diet Coke, sugar-free mints, and chewing gum and energy bars of every stripe. They are regulars at the Union Square Farmers' Market but also at Dylan's Candy Bar, the sweets emporium. They worship "eco-gastronomic" chef Alice Waters and commit to memory passages of books like *Eat This, Not That!* by Dave Zinczenko. But then they fall at the feet of the guru of the month like Tonya Zuckerbrot, of fibre cracker fame, and cleanse peddler Denise Mari, founder of Organic Avenue.

It is a strange cocktail of the good, the bad, and the horrendous: porridge for breakfast and half a can of cupcake frosting for lunch; a tuna burger and coleslaw at Union Square Café, then a week of tea made from lemon juice, maple syrup, and cayenne pepper. One woman I interviewed, who didn't want her name used, eats high-fibre bars every two hours, some lean protein, and not much else. Actress Julianne Moore, whom I've seen in yoga class, has a similar regimen of breakfast cereal, granola bars, and yogurt, according to an interview she gave to a women's magazine. The cheaters I interviewed live on Starbucks and energy drinks. They give up carbs and swear off fat. They keep bowls of boiled egg whites in their refrigerators and vats of mini Reese's Peanut Butter Cups in their cupboards.

My knee-jerk reaction to this kind of eating is nannyish finger wagging. Tsk! Tsk! Who wants to live that way? You're polluting your temple! But part of me is also, believe it or not, envious. How do they pull it off? These women eat terribly but look fantastic. Honestly, I don't have the discipline to do what many of them do. On Yom Kippur, the Jewish day of atonement, I rarely make it past noon with the required fasting. For the size 0s, 2s, and 4s (UK sizes 4, 6 and 8) I've been interviewing, swinging between deprivation and binging seems instinctive. As far as I can tell, they keep slimmer than their counterparts across the United States (who tip the scale at an average of twelve stone, according to the Centers for Disease Control) by throwing every nutritional rule ever written out the window. They skip a meal, snack late at night, gorge on refined sugar, and ignore entire food groups.

There is no shame in dieters falling off the wagon. We all do it. If there were no cheating, there would be no forty-billion-dollar (twenty-five-billion pound) weight-loss industry; no magazines like *Shape*, *Women's Health*, and *Women's Fitness*; no Splenda; and probably a lot fewer fish in the sea. When I say cheating, I mean eating in ways we're not "supposed" to. It is bigger than we are. There's even a cottage industry of diets based on the concept. *The Cheater's Diet* encourages strategies like having three drinks instead of four over a weekend and cutting back calories by 25 percent. *The Cheat to Lose Diet* manipulates carbs in an attempt to shed pounds. My favourite is *Cheat Your Way Thin*, which incorporates "cheat days" when you have licence to eat anything your taste buds desire.

As you probably know, diets tend not to work on a long-term basis. Most dieters regain more weight than they lost within four or five years. Some researchers even think dieting is a consistent predictor of future weight gain. In one study, both men and women who participated in formal weight-loss programmes gained significantly more weight over a two-year period than those who had not participated. My conclusion: no wonder we cheat on our diets! If dieting is futile, why bother sticking to the rules?

I have spent the last year talking to women I know about this topic—about food, eating habits, dieting tips, and weaknesses. I called everyone I know. I spoke to friends of friends and their friends. I approached any woman I could find who looked and seemed fit—even strangers on the street. My only agenda was to analyze patterns and understand a city's appetites. Although I made an effort to choose women who looked healthy—nice skin, shiny hair, visible muscle tone—oddly, in many conversations, I heard the same type of objections: "I have the worst diet," "I have a strange diet," or "You shouldn't talk to me; my diet is crazy."

Courtney is a good example. Courtney and I don't know each other well, but we worked together a few years ago at a magazine. Sitting in my office, I would watch her breeze through the halls, noting the men who swivelled to gawk in her wake. To look at Courtney, you wouldn't think: crazy eater. You'd think she was confident. She's a tall, gorgeous brunette with streaked hair, caramel eyes, and a waist smaller than the average man's hand span. She exuded competence, energy, well-being, and fitness.

Yet before we meet for lunch, Courtney warns me about her eating habits and how her friends chide her for them. Her warning turns out to be true. Her eating habits are not what you'd call conventional, and they haven't been for a long time. As our lunch begins, Courtney provides details from the fad diets she followed in high school. In one, she ate nothing but frozen yogurt. In another, she allowed herself only five grams of fat a day—about the amount you get in a teaspoon of olive oil.

Since then, her eating has improved, relatively speaking. About six years ago, Courtney came down with a bad cold and lost some weight. To keep it off, she decided she would cut out all carbs, which whittled another two stone from her frame. She says she hasn't had a carbohydrate since then. "Everyone was like, you're sick, what's wrong with you, your body is going to go into shock! But I found it was great for me. I could eat as much fat as I wanted. I haven't had pasta in six years. I'm the girl who when you pass the pizza pulls off the cheese and eats it."

In the arc of bad Manhattan eaters, Courtney certainly isn't the worst. When we meet, it's at a sushi restaurant, and she orders a tuna steak tartar and a salad. That's certainly respectable. But as she begins to list the particulars of her diet, I can't help worrying. She will have a bowl of berries and a banana, but not pineapple and not carrots. On occasion, she says, she will buy a chocolate chip cookie and pick out the chocolate bits, which are low in carbs, but she'll eat them with some crumbs clinging to them so she still gets the cookie flavour.

Last night she was meeting a friend at a bar after work at 6:30, so she stopped on the way at a convenience store and made a dinner of two sticks of string cheese and some watermelon. The melon, she says, helps you to lose weight and hydrates you at the same time. She limits the amount of wine she drinks and typically orders vodka, another low-carbohydrate trick. When I ask her if this way of eating is healthy, she tells me she gets that question all the time.

"People think I have a major problem with my eating. Just recently I've been getting really full. My friend was, like, because you have a severe eating disorder." She disagrees. "I don't have a disorder," she tells me. "I eat a lot. This is what I like to eat."

Personalized habits that work to keep women thin is how I think of this kind of eating strategy. I would like to emphasize these habits are unhealthy and that I don't like them, but I came across so many examples in my reporting that I thought it was as much a part of the Manhattan Diet as portion control and whole foods, brown rice, and spring greens. As I thought about "cheaters' little helpers," I started wondering if there were any lessons to be drawn from bad habits. Could cheating be a diet aid and not a source of dishonour?

The thought dogged me as I began to study my twenty-five volunteers' food journals. One of the first things I noticed was that their journals were uniformly un-diety, full—*full*—of red velvet cupcakes, marshmallow jelly beans, Reese's Peanut Butter Cups Minis, Gummy Bears, and Snickers Minis. That's what made their entries so refreshing to read. I didn't find myself wondering how it would be possible to eat that way or about all the work that went into their überhealthy meals. The journals felt honest. There were times, after cooking with their daughters, that women would simply eat a hunk of coffee cake as dinner, chased by a glass or two of wine. A long day at the office triggered a meal of French-bread pizza followed by apple pie with whipped cream followed by handfuls of Frosted Mini-Wheats.

I started to realize that there might be some wisdom here, that in their own way, these women might actually be on to something: eating badly is part of eating well. A chocolate bar or a handful of Skittles might not have any significant nutritional value, but psychologically, they're lifesavers. They taste good. They're what people eat. So instead of trying to ban or demonize them, just let them in. It's cheating, from the standard dieting point of view, but so what? To me, the beauty of the Manhattan Diet is that it reflects how a population of thin women eat. It's not a fad diet, it's a diet for life—a way of eating, not a prescription. You don't go on and off the Manhattan Diet, you just live it. Real women eat junk food, fattening food, "bad" food. It's okay.

Here is an example. This is a day from the diary of a woman in her mid-forties who works in the fashion industry. She is shapely and in shape, and she's very energetic, perhaps from all of the coffee and sugar she consumes. There are telltale signs of dieting: skimmed milk, hard-boiled eggs, cottage cheese. But she also rewards herself.

11 a.m.
     ½ chocolate chip cookie, 3 cappuccinos
1 p.m.
     1 scrambled egg made with butter
     1 slice cinnamon-raisin toast, buttered
2 p.m.
     125g pineapple cottage cheese
3 p.m.
     1 hard-boiled egg
     1 small skinny white mocha with just a touch of whipped
        cream from Starbucks
     10 baby carrots
4 p.m.
     1 small apple
5 p.m.
     ½ bagel with cream cheese

7:30 p.m.
> 15 tortilla chips with hummus

8 p.m.
> 175g rotisserie chicken with 1 teaspoon barbecue
> sauce
>
> 2 tablespoons mashed potatoes
>
> 6 tablespoons broccoli sautéed in olive oil and garlic salt

9:20 p.m.
> 1 small box raisins

This is what I mean by "cheating": allowing yourself to eat the things that people on diets aren't "supposed" to have. It's a diet strategy that indulges the "bad girl" who can't resist her treats. And it's totally healthy! No taboos! A lollipop at 4 p.m. isn't going to kill you and, God willing, it will keep you from a full-immersion Rocky Road ice cream binge at 2 a.m.

You may have noticed from my descriptions that the foods Manhattan ladies cheat with tend to be sugary, not fatty. So choose candy, not tortilla chips; cake, not french fries. As far as I can tell, it's all about the sweet tooth. I keep snack bags with 100-calorie portions of Gummy Bears (twelve), jelly beans (twenty-five), and peanut brittle (about 20 grams) in my cupboard. I'm allowed one portion in the afternoon. I also have a stash of Nips, a toffee like hard candy with a chocolate centre. They're 30 or so calories apiece and give my cocoa craving a rest. Uma Thurman is an M&M's freak, so you can go that route (twenty-five). Lots of women swear by dark chocolate; it kick-starts endorphin production, which gives you a feeling of pleasure, and contains serotonin, which acts as an antidepressant. It's hard to go wrong there, plus it passes muster with the "health police" in ways the other sweets don't.

There is actually scientific documentation to back up the theory that eating a regulated amount of sweets is good for you. One study, published in the *American Journal of Clinical Nutrition*, compared two groups: one that was overfed mostly carbohydrates and one that was overfed mostly fats. Conventional diet wisdom has it that carbs, in everything from pasta to bagels and brownies, are evil. But in this study, the carb loaders trumped the fat-eaters. The carb crowd stored just 75 percent of the calories they consumed, whereas the fat-eating group stored between 90 and 95 percent of the calories they consumed. What's more, the carbohydrate overeaters experienced a jump in carb oxidation and energy consumption.

A study published in the *International Journal of Obesity* looked at another method of dietary cheating: going over the top on a night out or with a special meal at home—for instance, fried chicken with mashed potatoes, gravy, rolls, and coleslaw, for a calorie count that could sustain a family of four. You may be surprised to learn, however, that it's a better dieting tactic to overeat than to undereat.

This study compared the metabolic rates of a group of overfed individuals and a group of fasters. After a day of being overfed, the so-called resting energy expenditure of the eaters jumped almost 9 percent. The people in this group burned up to 424 more calories than usual over the course of the following day. They even burned more calories while they were sleeping! And there was no significant weight gain. Meanwhile, the metabolisms of the people who fasted slowed to a crawl. Their twenty-four-hour resting energy expenditure *fell* 9 percent, and they burned 526 *fewer* calories than they had the day before.

Of course, you can't overeat like this every day, because then it's not merely cheating on a diet. It's a recipe for heart failure. The trick is figuring out how to cheat in a controlled way that lets you feel satisfied. Three skinny or whole milk lattes a day is probably too many. Cut back to one or even two. Nutritionist Sharon Richter doesn't forbid her clients to eat Tasti D-Lite, a non-dairy, low-cal version of frozen yogurt. She might suggest instead something like peanut butter, which you might think is fatty but which is actually good for you. Likewise, if she receives a text from a client in a Mexican restaurant asking about nachos or chimichurris, Richter will check out the menu online and steer the client towards dishes like ceviche or fajitas. "Anything is allowed," says Richter, but she adds that some cheats are safer than others.

The primary risk of the "controlled cheating" method is the stopping at one 100-calorie bag of jelly beans or one rasher of bacon. You just have to figure out which forbidden foods work for you. Richter suggests peanut butter as a substitute for candy or a frozen dessert. I can't have peanut butter in the house. If I do, I go for it with a spoon. I start by thinking, "This is okay, it's healthy." I eat it straight out of the jar—no bread, no crackers, no celery. But I can't stop at one or two spoonfuls. I stop at half a jar. Then I throw out the rest. Peanut butter might be healthier than chocolate or jelly beans, but not in 500-gram servings. So I don't buy it any more. I stick with candy, because with that I seem to have an off switch.

Like the ladies I interviewed, I also have a notable record as a fad dieter. My low point was in college when I went on a liquid protein diet, eating absolutely nothing for six weeks except a sticky, cherry-flavoured syrup that supposedly contained all of the protein and nutrients my body needed. I could drink water, coffee, and no-cal drinks, but I couldn't have any solids. I supposedly went into something called ketosis (in which the body burns fat for energy) and lost two stone.

That summer I worked as a waitress in a resort in the Poconos, gorging on french fries and milk shakes. My father says he can still remember the day I got off the plane in August, three stone heavier than the day he and my mom had sent me off. In photos from that period, I look like the "before" picture in a diet ad, with my shirt buttons straining and my trousers three sizes too small. In years to come I would try the Cabbage Soup Diet, the Baked Potato Diet, various self-concocted juice fasts, and fanatic calorie counting.

The 100-Calorie Candy Jar

Try keeping any *one* of these items around to snack on.

1 Drumstick or Chupa Chups lollipop

1 Cadbury Fudge Bar

6 squares Aero

1 Reese's Peanut Butter Cup

25 M&M's

3½ liquorice twists

25 Skittles

2 Twix Minis

5 Werther's Originals

4 Milky Way Minis

5 Starbursts

1 bag Jelly Tots

60 Smarties

1 bag Milky Way Magic Stars

2 squares dark chocolate

These days, my weight and my life have settled into a better routine—in no small part because I am in Manhattan. I have no idea what size or shape I might be had I gone back to Orlando to live, stayed in Syracuse after I graduated, or entered some other parallel health universe. Anyway, I now apply my fifty-plus years of eating experience in a more sane way than at any other point in my life. I cheat, too, mostly by skipping meals, putting too much sugar in my coffee, or drinking too much wine with dinner. But overall I am pretty happy with my balance of foods and my general health.

I've become a believer in real food, putting me squarely in the whole foods, whole grains camp.

Fad diets, meanwhile, are still with us. I have to say I was surprised by the legions of them circulating in my postcode. Almost without exception, the hundred or so women I interviewed had all dabbled in trendy dieting of one type or another, like the Eat for Breakfast What You Had for Dinner Diet, the Four-Hour Body Diet, the Paleo Diet, the Cabbage Soup Diet, the Popcorn Diet, or the Blood-Type Diet. Many had been on, or were still on, Weight Watchers, which isn't a fad but has become faddish in Manhattan in the last few years, especially among fashion types. As far as I can tell, the appeal of these diets seems to be as much in the community they create as the results they promise. "You're on the Flat Belly Diet? Me, too!" It's a bonding exercise. In some instances, the diets are a kind of entertainment.

That's at least how Melanie Dunea describes her diet addiction. In general, the five-foot-five, forty-year-old photographer eats pretty well. When her weight rises past nine stone, she reverts to fruit and yogurt in the morning, skips pastries, keeps lunch and dinner light, and cuts back on salt, sugar, and wine. But given her work and travel schedule—she is often on the road for weeks at a time shooting celebrity subjects like Taylor Swift, Andie MacDowell, and Steve Martin—she also likes the discipline and fast results of a fad diet. Being up on the latest diet has its own currency, too. If the celebrities are on a particular diet, you want to check it out. "It's a little harmless fun," she tells me.

Most recently, Melanie attempted the Master Cleanse, a regimen that involves drinking a tea made from water, maple syrup, lemon juice, and cayenne pepper for ten days. Celebrities like Beyoncé and Gwyneth Paltrow have helped repopularize the Cleanse, which dates back to the 1940s and has wafted in and out of style since then. My college-era liquid protein diet would qualify as a cleanse, too, I guess, as would the other daylong fasts I've concocted. From what I've read, Beyoncé peeled off one and a half stone in ten days on the Master Cleanse, preparing for her role as the lithe Deena Jones in *Dreamgirls*. Paltrow has written about the benefits of cleansing on her blog, *Goop*. Melanie says she tried it "for the challenge and the purification. I like being told what to eat." Although she was happy with the results—"I think it's fabulous," she tells me—not everyone she knows was so impressed. "My trainer quit me," Melanie confides. "She said it was unhealthy and didn't want to work with me any more."

Cleansing is so popular in Manhattan that it warranted a front-page story in the Fashion and Style section of the *New York Times*. The reporter, in her late forties and trying to lose one and a half stone, noted that juices and juice-cleanse companies are "as ubiquitous at Fashion Week events as cigarettes and Adderall." She tried the BluePrintCleanse, but there are many others, including Organic Avenue and the CoolerCleanse.

Each owes its celebrity at least partly to a famous dieter. Before Paltrow wrote about Organic Avenue on her blog, it was an under-the-radar operation catering to vegans and yogis who wanted a juice fast. Afterwards, actresses Eva Mendes, Liv Tyler, and Naomi Watts materialized in photos, drinking Organic Avenue products. BluePrintCleanse has good names behind it, too, including the designer Jason Wu, who says he cleanses with the product one or two days a week because he "forgets to eat." Sarah Jessica Parker has also been snapped in photos toting a bottle of BluePrint-Cleanse. The draw for CoolerCleanse is actress Salma Hayek, a cofounder of the company.

Given New York's love affair with Whole Foods, whole grains, and locally grown anything, it was inevitable that diet marketeers would try and tap into that mind-set. Whereas I was told in 1977 that fasting would make me skinny, today's cleansers are told they will "detox," have clearer skin, have more energy, and feel "cleaner." The inference, I suppose, is that our kidneys and livers need help in doing their jobs. Weight loss isn't mentioned, although it's the only reason, aside from a religious practice, that anyone would go through the ordeal of fasting.

The programmes cost in the neighbourhood of $65 (£40) a day, surely producing some of the most expensive pee in the country. Pass by morning drop-off at an Upper East Side private school, and half the moms will be toting their BluePrintCleanse bags with a day's worth of juices. Ditto the offices of some fashion magazines. You can also have your six-juice allotment delivered to your home or office by rickshaw. As for the taste, the *New York Times* reporter wrote, "Here's the thing. That green juice? It was like drinking everything bad that ever happened to me in high school."

The websites for these products tout their health benefits and quote doctors who vouch for cleansing (eliminate Lupus! Eczema!). But there is little or no scientific data indicating that we need cleansing plans or that they are helpful, says Kim Diamond, a nutritionist and trainer who works with executives from the Sony Corporation. "A healthy body is very good at cleansing itself—the kidneys, liver, and GI (gastrointestinal) tract effectively and efficiently remove toxins," she says. And the possible side effects sound like a parody of one of those television drug commercials: fatigue, hunger, constipation, headaches, and irritability. Repeated fasts could result in vitamin deficiencies, muscle breakdown, blood-sugar problems, and weakening of the immune system.

Yet the risks don't deter the determined. Novelist Tatiana Boncompagni admits that her BluePrintCleanse experience was initially torturous, but then she got hooked. "There was a psychological connection to how I felt. It did fantastic things to my body. I lost weight. My skin looked great. If you are eating a lot of sugar, you don't taste your food. After a juice fast, it allows you to reset your taste buds, and you realize enough energy to get through the day. It's very calming; it became a meditative, calming experience."

Now she cleanses regularly. And she looks gorgeous.

Manhattan Diet Secrets

- *Depriving yourself of something only makes you want it more.* Instead of creating taboos, figure out a way to incorporate them into your diet in a controlled way. Keep bags of 100-calorie sugar rushes on hand, such as jelly beans or chocolate-covered raisins. But learn to eat just one bag.

- *Substitute-cheat.* If you're mainlining 500 grams of frozen yoghurt because it's low-cal, try a smaller portion of the real thing: ice cream. You might like it better, and it will be more filling.

- *Acknowledge your weaknesses.* If you really can't control yourself around a particular food—it's peanut butter for me—don't buy it. Try something else, like sunflower seeds or pistachios, that don't make you crazy.

- *Not even Beyoncé is big on the Master Cleanse any more.* She has said in interviews that she gained the weight back right after *Dreamgirls* and that she wouldn't recommend cleansing to anyone, especially someone who's not trying to lose weight for a movie.

- *If you insist on fasting and have $65 (£40) a day to blow,* a 1,200-calorie juice fast probably won't hurt you over a short period (a day or two), but definitely don't cleanse repeatedly, and do it only under the care of a nutritionist or a doctor.

9

Expert Handling
How We Get Help

When most women want to lose weight or get in shape, they buy the latest diet book, join a gym, or sign up for a Zumba class. Some try power yoga or count calories. Others look for group support in programmes like Weight Watchers or Jenny Craig.

Manhattan women do all of that. And then they open their wallets.

These women hire personal chefs and strength trainers, massage therapists and dietitians. New moms firm their cores with private Pilates instructors and jump-start their metabolisms with one-to-one Spin classes. Runners turn to Olympic coaches. Golfers hire pros. Some women track down a celebrity trainer like Tracy Anderson or Kacy Duke, and others go with entourages. When film publicist Peggy Siegal celebrated her sixtieth birthday at the Plaza

Athenee, she distributed a booklet with the names and contact information of twenty-three experts she credited with helping her look so fantastic, according to press reports at the time. (Among those named: Richard Frankel, noted for great "toe reductions"; Roy Geronemus, a dermatologist who lasers off sun spots; nutritionist Jordan Carroll; and Rich Cardone, a masseur.)

Overkill? Or best practices? To be honest, it's a little of both. No one really *needs* a team of experts to achieve Kelly Ripa abs—or really *needs* Kelly Ripa abs, for that matter. Yet the women of Manhattan really want to look good. It's a priority for them. Fitness pros are just another personal-maintenance line item, like a weekly mani-pedi or a Brazilian Blowout hair-straightening treatment. They're considered part of good grooming. They're efficient, and they're what everyone else is doing.

Of course, the $100-an-hour (£60) Pilates guru, the $150-an-hour (£90) private chef, and the $90-an-hour (£55) osteopath add up—in some cases to the tune of $30,000 (£18,000) a year. Are they totally necessary? Probably not. But when you've got the money, cost becomes secondary. It's not about the cash; it's about going the distance, which in New York is defined as help. Worried that your preschooler is an underachiever? Bring on a tutor. Must run the marathon? Get a running coach. It's the same principle.

Unless you're a professional athlete or planning to be one, this reliance on pros might seem a little excessive—self-absorbed and self-indulgent. Of course, it's not as though New Yorkers are alone in this mania. Plenty of other fitness-crazed metropolises boast armies of health and fitness experts. It's just that in the more sensible heartland, you'd be hard-pressed to find more than a few pro clusters in any given town. I know; I tried.

I started by Googling Pilates instructors in Jackson, Mississippi, a city of 175,000 or so. I found three names for the whole city. How about a nutritionist or a dietitian in my hometown suburb of Maitland, Florida (population 14,000)? I consulted Dietician.com's expert locator and uncovered—zero. Looking for a sports chiropractor in Three Rivers, California (population 2,358), where my friend Chris lives, rides horses, and could use said services? The closest chiropractor of any kind is almost 130 miles away, in Los Banos, California. Yet conducting the same search in my backyard in Manhattan produced pages and pages of listings. I couldn't begin to quantify them. Thousands? I know one nutritionist who lives two floors above me. For all I know, there are three Pilates instructors up there, too.

It's not surprising that the experts flock here. It's where the work is. But the flip side of the coin is that all that namby-pamby hand-holding actually produces results. Let's say, for argument's sake, that all of these trainer-addicted Manhattanites gave up their experts cold turkey and tried to stay in shape on their own. More than likely, they'd flame out. In the absence of a personal trainer or a nutritionist, most dieters and exercisers quit.

A study of commercial weight-reduction programmes (Jenny Craig and Weight Watchers) showed that half of the participants dropped out after six weeks; after twelve weeks, the dropout rate was 70 percent. Typically, gyms lose a third or more of their members every year, and some lose as many as half. The reasons aren't that hard to figure out: inertia, loss of momentum, and the scariness of letting go of old habits. With a trainer, a nutritionist, or some other pro, you have fewer excuses. You have a private cheerleader holding your hand through the rough spots.

The difference with a one-to-one expert is what cable network exec Cristina Cuomo refers to as the "kick my butt" factor. Trainers don't let you wimp out on the fifth set of repetitions, sneak out of class before it's over, or give you a pass to stay at home instead of hitting the gym. They're motivated when you're not—they want to get paid, after all—and produce results for their clients. The opposite is, presumably, also true, since you're paying for the services, and want to get your money's worth—not unlike psychotherapy. It turns out that everyone needs a little in the way of external incentives.

I will hold Cristina up as an example. She happens to be one of the faces you see in New York gossip columns and on fashion-orientated websites, like Style.com and Newyorksocialdiary.com. She is married to *Good Morning America* anchor Chris Cuomo (the brother of the current governor of New York) and pals around with other lovelies, such as Fernanda Niven, the granddaughter of actor David Niven. In Cristina's circles, healthy, raw, and organic foods are big topics. So are exercise and working out. Her husband has blogged about training for a triathlon and has chronicled on air his effort to shed 10 pounds. Her friend Fernanda is an investor in Organic Avenue, the raw foods and cleanse company. Cristina herself is a former high school athlete, and at forty-one she still has that hale, lacrosse-girl, private school polish about her (she was actually captain of the hockey and tennis teams and a state fencing champion).

The day we meet for lunch, she looks fantastically fit, as though nothing bad has ever entered her body. In fact, she tells me, she grew up in a presciently health-conscious New York family in which her mom made yogurt from scratch and served organic everything. Her mother had her so well-trained that one of the early differences Cristina had with her husband, Chris, was over organic chicken. He said it was scrawny and tasteless. She said a conventional bird was fatty. They settled with a cook-off. Cristina won, and the family now eats organic only.

Cristina was a little sulky after the birth of her third child when her weight didn't magically melt back to nine stone, the way it had after babies one and two. She had a tyre around her middle and was sluggish. She was running, but that wasn't taking the weight off fast enough, and it wasn't giving her the sculpted, defined look she wanted. She got stuck on the thought that the body you have at forty is the body you'll have for the rest of your life, and suddenly she wanted results yesterday. "I was still nursing, but I thought, 'Shit, I have to get into shape.'"

Cristina tracked down a trainer and signed up for three days a week. The two worked on sculpting and firming and making her "feel comfortable in a bathing suit again." On alternate days, Cristina went to Spin classes. She changed her diet. Within three months, she was in the shape she wanted to be in. On her own, Cristina says, she never would have been that disciplined. "I needed someone to mould me into the person I wanted to be."

I'm not sure I would describe Cristina as a slacker. Yet even she felt the need for a trainer. No magic there. Hard work produced measurable results. Team up with any fitness expert, and you're likely to get similar results—much more so than if you go it solo. A study published in the *Annals of Internal Medicine* followed three hundred dieters, some of whom worked with a registered dietitian by e-mail or by phone, some who met with a dietitian in person, and some who went solo, with no outside counselling. The dieters all cut their calories, exercised, set weight goals, and used the appetite-suppressant medication sibutramine.

Guess what? There was a direct correlation between counselling and weight loss. The more help the participants got, the more weight they lost. Those in the self-help group lost on average 5.2 percent of their original body weight. The group with e-mail support from a registered dietitian lost a little more: 5.9% of their body weight. The people who chatted with a dietitian on the phone dropped 7.7% of their body weight, and the group that met the diet pro in person registered an 8.9 percent weight loss.

The help you get doesn't even need to be one-to-one expertise. A study done at the University of Minnesota in Minneapolis showed that dieters who regularly attended weight-loss classes shaved off more pounds in eleven weeks than those who skipped class. This isn't incontrovertible proof: there are lots of reasons people skip class. But there's no arguing with the motivation of a class setting. It's the reason exercise chains like Equinox, New York Health & Racquet Club, Exhale, and Crunch thrive.

How They Diet

GWYNETH PALTROW

The actress is clean as a whistle. She is famous for fasting a couple of times a year—including with the hardcore Master Cleanse, which she describes as "not pretty." She has her own detox doctor, Alejandro Junger. She's written about the custom cleanses Junger has created for her and has run excerpts from his book on her blog, *Goop*.

I learned about the efficacy of the pros in a less clinical way when I developed a huge crush on my yoga teacher. It was during my hard-core Ashtanga phase, about ten years ago, premotherhood. Ashtanga is a gruelling but gratifying yoga practice in which you execute a set series of challenging poses at a pretty fast clip, sweating a lot in the process. In addition to having the stamina of Rahm Emanuel, you also have to have a core so tight you can spring onto your feet from a backbend. You also have to be able to get into a backbend. I was having trouble with both parts—and with about half of the other poses, too. To get up to speed, I started taking private lessons at home with my teacher, the brilliant Eric Powell.

Eric would arrive at my apartment, we'd go through the poses, and he would "adjust" me into the proper positions. I'm thinking of the hip opener, *baddha konasana*. In that pose, you sit on the floor with the soles of your feet together and your knees falling out to the side. You then bend over and graze the floor with your forehead. It's something I imagine comes easily to eight-year-olds and ballet dancers. Your knees are supposed to actually touch the floor, but mine were a few inches away. So Eric did the natural thing: he stood on my thighs until there was parquet-to-knee contact, and I gasped in pain. In another position, *prasarita podottanasana*, I stood with my legs wide apart, bent over from the waist until my head touched the floor. Then Eric would take my hands, which were clasped together behind my back, and wrench my arms over my head until they touched the ground, too.

The more Eric pulled and pushed and twisted me, the more I looked forward to our sessions. It was the Stockholm syndrome, yogi style. I was enthralled. I wanted to please him. I wanted to be his star student. I started inviting him to do things: come to dinner parties, go to concerts. He always said no. But I kept asking. And I was hardly alone. There were about ten other women in the gym's Ashtanga class with me, and we all were in yoga love with Eric. We were also, I'm sure, at the most limber, strongest points of our lives. At least I was, and I owed this equally to Eric's talents as a teacher and my forty-year-old hormones.

Thinking back on that time, I realize it makes perfect sense. When you're working that physically close to someone, you can't help but bond. You're exercising with someone who is pretty much a perfect physical specimen. If Eric had a superfluous gram of body fat, I couldn't see it. He could hold a handstand for longer than I stay in *shavasana* (the corpse pose). He hopped forward from downward dog in balletic slow motion. It would have been embarrassing not to try my absolute hardest with that example in the room.

Granted, the whole expert crush thing can spin out of control. One day you're working with a trainer. The next thing you know, you're signing up for weekly boot camp so that you will have more staying power for your trainer. Then you add yoga, then Spin three times a week. It's kind of like the woman who cleans her house before the housekeeper arrives. Before you know it, you're exercising every day and you've lost control of your schedule, which perhaps isn't all that much of an issue. Fifty-one percent of women in a *Fitness* magazine survey said they'd skip sex for a year if it meant they'd be skinny. If they'd happily sacrifice sex, perhaps giving up their free time is no biggie.

The Manhattan Fitness Firmament

Here are a few of the more in-demand fitness and diet experts in New York City. Anderson, McGee, and Pettijohn also work in other places.

Tracy Anderson: She's the fitness trainer who Gwyneth Paltrow and Madonna built up. Thanks to Paltrow's endless promotion in particular, Anderson has garnered a large following in New York and around the country. Paltrow is reportedly a partner in Anderson's $900/(£500) per month Tribeca gym (initiation fees are separate), where gals line up to achieve the long and lean look Anderson is known for. For you West Coasters, there's a Los Angeles branch, too.

Jordan Carroll: She has retaught much of the Upper East Side how to eat. Carroll has her clients write down every gram of fat they eat for two weeks, then comes up with a personalized plan. It's all very healthy. No tricks, just lots of protein and fresh fruits and vegetables. You don't skip meals.

Stacey Griffith: She's a celebrity Spin instructor affiliated with the Soul Cycle studios. Back in her Hollywood days, Stacey worked with actresses like Brooke Shields and Nicole Kidman. Now she's catering to New York's fit elite.

Kristin McGee: She's a private yoga and Pilates instructor with clients like Steven Martin, Tina Fey, and Bethenny Frankel. If you can't afford one-to-one sessions, Kristin teaches a few group classes at Equinox and Reebok.

Jill Pettijohn: Jill is a nurse from New Zealand who moved from waitressing to having her own catering company to cooking privately for celeb clients like Donna Karan, Tom Cruise, Drew Barrymore, and Steven Seagal. She is a vegetarian and leads raw-food seminars in places like Bali.

At that point, we're in obsession territory. Price is no object. Time is no object. Nothing is an object. Women who hire three, four, five, or more experts to ensure they excel in every part of their health and fitness routine are a small minority, but in New York, not *that* small. Many pros I spoke to told me their clients often have teams of experts to advise them on everything from their golf swing to weight management to black diamond (an advanced ski trail) technique. They're the outliers who are setting an example for other women to follow. They might describe themselves as perfectionists—or, if they have a sense of humour, extremists.

Tina Basle is a little of both. The thirty-thousand-dollar-a-year expert tab I mentioned at the beginning of this chapter belongs to Tina, a forty-four-year-old amateur marathoner I met through her trainer, Gordon Bakoulis. Tina came to running rather late, taking up the sport in 2005 at the urging of her boyfriend. Within a year, she had run a marathon, then she did a few more. When she pulled a hamstring in 2009 training for the Chicago marathon, she didn't think much about it. Instead of resting, she just kept running—until one day, when she couldn't run any more because the muscle was so seriously damaged.

That still didn't stop her. During the next two years, Tina began gearing up to race again, this time with the help of a team of experts. She started by consulting with a sports chiropractor a couple of times a week. Then she added a twice-a-week private Pilates instructor. Then she hired Ms. Bakoulis, a well-known local running coach who herself had made the Olympic trials five times. To round out the entourage, Tina also brought on board a massage therapist.

"I don't know," she says. "Maybe that's what it takes for a forty-four-year-old to run a marathon."

Price didn't really factor into the equation. In Tina's mind, it was all about getting back in the game. When she breaks down the costs for me, pro by pro, I'm a little taken aback: the Pilates teacher is $100 (£70) an hour, the chiropractor is $175 (£100) a session (depending on where she is in her insurance cycle), the weekly massage therapist is $70 (£45) an hour, and Bakoulis, the running coach, is $80 (£50) a month (they mostly just communicate by e-mail). By my estimates, Tina is shelling out about $2,500 (£1,500) a month, at least before her deductible has been covered. It's not something she worries about too much, though. After all, no one forced her to staff up after the injury. She was just determined to enter another marathon. "I didn't quit running," she says. "I got the entourage."

Tina's extreme commitment brings to mind something I was told by Heather Bauer, a nutritionist. She says she has almost no obese clients and few overweight ones. "Most of the people I work with usually just need to lose 5 to 10 pounds," says Bauer. "Anywhere else in the country, they'd be considered thin." It's an observation I heard again and again, and it puts my Manhattan demographic in perspective. Even though my subjects primarily cited lack of motivation as an explanation for using the pros, it is a bit of a misnomer. They are *very* motivated. For the most part, they are already fit and slim and are just looking for ways to get even more so, or to get back on the wagon if they've somehow slipped off.

The bottom line is that using a pro is easier than doing it yourself. Pros work around your schedule. They come up with variations on meals and exercises so you don't have to. They push you. When your life is crammed full of other things, the experts relieve some of the burden. They worry about your fitness for you. That's their job, says Kim Diamond, the nutritionist and trainer who oversees the corporate wellness programme at Sony USA. "When people come in to see me, they always say the same thing: 'Tell me what to do, Kim. Tell me what to eat.'" So that's what she does. She makes the decisions. There's always the risk that you'll end up with a lousy trainer or nutritionist who steers you in the wrong direction or gives bad advice. But mostly, there's no downside, except for having to spend all that money.

Manhattan Diet Secrets

- *You don't* need *an expert to help you shape up*. But you might need someone to kick your butt. With the help of experts, you will be more inspired and get faster results than without them. They're worth every penny you can spare.

- *Suppose you can't spare a lot of pennies on private coaches.* There are lots of ways to save. Kim Diamond suggests working with clients for half an hour instead of an hour. You can keep going on your own for another half an hour after you're done with the one-to-one training, so that two half-hour sessions feel almost the same as two hour-long ones. You can also team up with friends for semi-private sessions, hire a trainer who's in training, and book the pros in their off-hours.

- *Getting a crush on your trainer is not a bad thing.* You will work harder and get faster results, and it makes working out all the more interesting. (Just don't act on those hormone-induced impulses.)

- *If one expert works wonders, imagine what two, three, or four can do.* You too might be able to run a marathon. Supplement visits to live pros with virtual ones. At sites like ExerciseTV.com, you can download videos from specific trainers for a small fee (99 cents to $2.99/70p to £1.85). Sites like Dailyom.com offer yoga programmes for which you pay what you can afford or think is appropriate.

- *Do your due diligence before you hire a specialist.* Make sure that he or she is qualified and comes with recommendations. When Sony senior director Lisa Gephardt worked with a staff trainer at a chain gym in Manhattan, he set her up with a cookie-cutter routine that was fine for a college frat boy but not so good for an injury-prone woman in her mid-thirties. Lisa ended up seriously hurting her shoulder. Now she is working with a trainer who has custom-designed a twice-a-week workout for her. "We're partners," she says of the new pro.

10

Confident in the Kitchen
How We Cook

My friend Myriam is standing in what she calls her "one-butt" kitchen, a phrase I believe is self-explanatory. The room measures about six feet by four feet on a good day like today, when there isn't a bag of groceries, her young daughter, or a footstool taking up space. In one corner is a four-burner stove with rings so close together you can cook on only three of them at a time. The countertop, if it weren't crammed with spices, napkins, dish soap, receipts, and other detritus, would be just big enough to accommodate a regulation-size cutting board. But cluttered it is, so instead there is a notebook-sized slab of wood. Myriam owns just a few cooking utensils—a grater, a chef's knife, and a wooden spoon—because there is no place to store anything else. She doesn't have a food processor, a blender, a toaster, or a microwave, for the same reason. Nor is there a dishwasher. Her favourite pot is fitted with a mesh basket on top so she can boil and steam simultaneously.

But really, who needs space? When I wrote *Diary of a Tuscan Chef*—a cookbook about Cesare's childhood—I tested 150 recipes in a kitchen exactly this size. It had the same tiny range and floor space. Myriam thinks nothing of throwing a dinner party for six that stars filet mignon in a morel reduction sauce, green beans almandine, and baked potatoes. Last night, she whipped up a rack of lamb for herself, her husband, and her daughter. The night before, it was coq au vin.

At the moment, she is pulling together a late lunch, an Iberico ham and mozzarella omelette, half of which she will save for her dinner. A melancholy Yves Montand is serenading us. (Myriam is French.) Her apartment is small, but it has soaring ceilings and lots of light. There are framed posters from French films on the walls, lending a garret-on-the-Seine vibe. The music, she tells me, transports her so that she feels like cooking, and I believe her. The mood is so soigné, it makes *me* feel like cooking.

I watch as my friend tosses chunks of onion into rapeseed oil. In a separate bowl, she mixes four eggs, some single cream, and salt and pepper. To the degree that there is room to do so, I start poking around. Myriam's refrigerator is stuffed, and it pops open at the touch. Each nook and cranny is spoken for, packed with bars of butter and cream cheese, an oily bundle of hand-cut smoked salmon, and a half-eaten tin of sardines. Cholesterol is clearly not an issue in this household. There's American, string, mozzarella, and cheddar cheese as well as three cartons of single cream. I see five different types of fruit and a few kinds of lettuce. There is a tub of hummus, carrots, onions, celery, and vegetables of every stripe. Even before Myriam tells me she shops every day, I can see that she does. The produce looks just-picked. It's a cook's refrigerator—someone who is hooked on seasonal ingredients and not shy about spending money on them.

Because Myriam was born in France, she has a bit of an advantage over your average home chef. She spent her early years shadowing an aunt who liked to whip up buttery escargot or frogs in garlic and coriander for dinner. Entering the kitchen was an adventure. Now she is one of those pleasure-deriving, fat-embracing European eaters. Her portions are small, but she savours, and throughout the day she keeps going with foods that scare most dieters: nuts, cheese, smoked salmon, and single cream that pack her refrigerator.

Her theory about eating is simple: it can't be a fixation. If it is, you'll always overeat. At forty-five years old and five feet four, Myriam tips the scale at just over eight stone. She's an elementary school science teacher who looks like a college coed. My dad, who is normally a tough sell, asks me how Myriam is doing almost every time we talk. That is in no small part, I'm sure, because of her girlish figure.

Here's what I think is Myriam's secret: she adores cooking. *Adores* it. She not only shops for food every day, she cooks every day, and with the exception of an occasional roasted chicken when she's exhausted, she almost never orders take-out. Although the restaurant delivery industry feeds thousands of Manhattan families, Myriam's family is not one of them. That food is greasy and suspicious, Myriam tells me. "Who knows what goes in there?" In contrast, when you cook for yourself, she says, "It feels good. There is a sense you are having food food. I sauté, I stir-fry. I know what kind of meat I'm using. I know what's in there."

If I had to name the biggest surprise I found in researching this book, it would be how much cooking slender people do. I just assumed it would be the opposite, that they'd be snipping open a bag of organic mixed salad leaves and dumping a can of water-packed tuna on top or ordering plain steamed Chinese vegetables and brown rice from the take-out place around the corner. I didn't see why New Yorkers would be any different from time-pressed cooking-phobes across the country. You certainly know about these Americans and might even be one: the growing population that is venturing into the kitchen to experiment less and less, even as it eats more and more; people who don't care about what they eat or who have more important things on their plates, so to speak.

From what I've read, half of Americans who eat at home rely on fast food, delivery, or takeout from restaurants or delis. If things keep going this way, I predict that ovens will soon be vestigial, like tonsils, with no useful function at all—except maybe to store sweaters and shoes. Already, a quarter of home meals made in 2009 were simply zapped in a microwave. That's more than double the percentage in 1985, according to the market research firm NPD. In a survey by the Pew Research Center, 68 percent of respondents said they couldn't live without a microwave—more than couldn't survive without a television, a computer, or a cell phone!

Meanwhile, the use of cooktops and stoves is decreasing, with only one-third of home meals prepared on those appliances, down from a little more than half in 1985. We're not even bothering with salads. In 1984, 22 percent of all in-home dinners included a salad; today it's just 16 percent.

Not so New York City. In this hotbed of chef worship and loca-vore piety, people are actually cooking *more* than they used to. When Zagat, the chronicler of all things foodie, surveyed 6,800 locals in 2009, two-thirds of them said that was the case. Of those Zagat questioned, some 60 percent said they were starting from scratch when they made a meal, not relying on prepared foods. Some of that newfound kitchen zeal can be chalked up to the era's down economy, but a lot of it is just constitutional.

Temperamentally, Manhattanites are tied to their apron strings. They are into food, into eating, and into cooking. They aspire to be chefs like Mario Batali, or at least Rachael Ray. Manhattanites support more grocery stores per capita than any other population in the country—a supermarket for every 4,800 residents—not to mention a mini-village of appliance speciality stores, where you can pick up everything from a potato ricer to a pizza screen. This is a town where the *New York Times*'s most e-mailed article might be a recipe for wholemeal pancakes or no-knead bread. The paper's "most popular story ever" list includes a recipe for ramen noodles with salty packet sauce.

Cooking is such a big part of the Manhattan lifestyle that it's a cultural litmus test in some circles. This plays out in the craze for trophy kitchens, even among those who don't cook: the Garland range, the Sub-Zero refrigerator, the Gaggia espresso machine. Stagnating economy or not, these appliances still hold sway. Actress Jess Hecht and her husband recently bought a new apartment with a tiny kitchen and are starting to renovate and enlarge it. Jess is big on home cooking but has found the process a bit unnerving, with the world sitting in judgement on her appliance and cabinet choices.

"If your architect says to you, 'Do you cook?', what is he asking really? "she wonders." Is he asking, 'Do you cook *well*?' Or 'Do you really *need* a six-burner stove?' Or is he asking, 'Do you just cook the standard dinner?' Everyone has these beautiful kitchens in New York, but they're still so busy making money for the next renovation that they don't use them."

To be sure, not every svelte New Yorker knows what to do with a mandoline, and plenty wouldn't know a pilot light from aviation hero Sully Sullenberger. I am friendly with quite a few locals who use their ovens for sweater and shoe storage. One of my cousins, who never eats at home, came close to selling her dining room a few years back. A family in an adjacent apartment wanted to convert the space into a nursery for a new baby. (The co-op board blocked the sale.) Others eat whatever is available. That might be a bowl of Cheerios with semi-skimmed milk or a couple of protein bars, while their kids get hot dogs or chicken nuggets.

But I am not so interested in that subset of thin. I am focusing on hard-core eaters who are thin both because they seem to be genetically predisposed to it and because they work at it in a healthy, realistic way. For these Manhattan ladies, cooking is core. Myriam makes dinner from scratch every night. Ditto for Theresa Passarelli, the ingredient-crazed mom who grew up in Brooklyn, my journalist friend Lauren Lipton, novelist Tatiana Boncompagni, and dozens of others I interviewed.

For those who don't have the mental capacity, time, patience, or inclination to cook like that daily, there are ways to compress the time and the strategies. Just read on, and remember that from a health and nutrition point of view, cooking at home beats dining out every time. It's not too hard to figure out why. Dine out, and you're at the whim of the chef, whose goals don't dovetail with yours.

"In a restaurant, it's about making money," says Tim Shaw, an instructor at the International Culinary Center and an adjunct professor in food studies at New York University. "It's not about your health. Even if you can afford Per Se every night, should you be eating pork belly that often?" he asks rhetorically. Chefs have to satisfy investors, critics, and suppliers. You, a health-conscious customer, come last. Instead, at home, you answer to you. "You have control over what you put in your food," says Shaw. You decide if you end up "with a 2,800-calorie main course with fifty-eight grams of fat."

This is one of the major reasons I prefer to eat in. I'm a decent, not a great, cook, but I am a calorie freak, much to Cesare's dismay. He'd eat out every night if he could. I find it a little stressful sometimes. There's too much emotional jujitsu. What should I order? What should I avoid? How much olive oil is in that dish? How much butter? At home, I know exactly what goes into everything.

I'm not saying I don't like to eat well. I do. I just like clean, simple delicious food. Since Cesare works most nights, my typical dinner with our daughter is pasta with roasted vegetables or a pork chop sautéed in olive oil, garlic, and rosemary. Sometimes I will deglaze the pan with some white wine or lemon juice, but that's as fancy as I get. It takes about ten minutes total. As I said, fast, simple, good, and healthy.

The New York cooks I interviewed are making dinner in a similar fashion. They're throwing together pasta, sausage, and broccoli;

making turkey tacos; or having a steak and a salad or a quick soup. Some, like Nancy Farkas, a lawyer, have shortcuts. She will use a premarinated steak or a piece of fish that she bought at the grocery store. All she does is grill her choice and pair it with a salad of pre-washed greens. That is an especially good strategy if you like variety in your diet. As you probably know, grocery stores sell premarinated meats in all flavours: Korean sesame, lime and cumin, or chilli and garlic. Just cook, add a glass of wine, and hey presto, you've got dinner. Gillie Holme, an artist and a chef, will make a pot of lentils that start as a soup on Sunday, morph into a salad on Monday, and become dinner with a fried egg on top on the third night.

What my women are *not* serving is processed food. Well, there might be a few organic burritos, macaroni and cheese ready meals, and a couple of veggie burgers. But there's no Lean Cuisine, no instant rice or noodles, and not even a frozen pizza. In the twenty-five diet diaries that I collected and studied, I found only a handful of dinners that involved packaged or even take-out food. There were quite a few restaurant meals and things like English muffins and some breakfast cereals, but when my dieters were home, they usually were cooking.

I think this is, in part, a demographic phenomenon. These are upwardly mobile, environmentally conscious gals for whom whole foods are an article of faith. They simply don't patronize Subway, Kentucky Fried Chicken, or Burger King. Their idea of fast food is a Starbucks cappuccino. On the day I am writing this, the Food and Drug Administration has just released new nutritional guide-lines, which among other things recommend that half the dinner plate should be occupied by vegetables and fruit and that people should eat less pizza and dessert. These aren't suggestions that apply to my people. They *already* cook and eat that way. It is part of Manhattan life in the fast lane, a declaration of political correct-ness and personal competency.

"New Yorkers want to do the best of the best and go as far as we can go," says Jodie Patterson, a home cook and the owner of a popular hair and beauty salon. "If you live in New York, you just get up and do. You have a certain level of confidence." She connects the dots to diet and cooking. "If I can be really healthy, it's one step closer to the goal of being the best." Jodie doesn't buy any prepared foods, and she uses only brown rice and organic fruits and vegetables.

We are chatting in her salon, Georgia, a laid-back, artfully curated spot around the corner from Daniel Boulud's trendy DBGB Kitchen and Bar and next door to Keith McNally's Pulino's Bar and Pizzeria. I mention the restaurant coordinates because they define the neighbourhood: trendy, good-looking, flush, with a pretence of raffishness. And they say something about Jodie, who before she opened her shop did fashion PR for designers like Zac Posen and Sean Jean. If you are interested in fashion and nightlife and the Manhattan scene, this is the right address.

Talking to Jodie is a trip. She is both calm and ambitious, two qualities I've always considered mutually exclusive. She also glows, radiating health. I listen to her serenely recount everything she's done in the last twenty-four hours, and I am not sure how she does it.

The saga starts with tending to her four-year-old, who was up all night with a fever and diarrhoea. After not sleeping—and nursing her youngest baby every few hours—Jodie packed up all four kids and took them to the hospital at 7:30 a.m., then after the visit, took the healthy ones to school, leaving the youngest with a babysitter. She took care of some routine business at the shop, then ended her day at 6 p.m., when she closed the salon, went home, and, with the babysitter, made dinner. The menu: grilled trout, spring greens, and rice and beans. She bathed the children and got them ready for bed, reading two books to each child. Then she had her own dinner and worked until she fell asleep. Today has been less hectic, but tonight she will attend two events, including a fundraiser with designer Michael Kors for the Dance Theater of Harlem.

The point of all this is the trout, spring greens, and rice and beans. It is fantastically healthy and, with planning, hardly a time drain. If you keep cooked brown rice and beans on hand (and you should), then you just have to grill the trout, which takes about twenty minutes. I have a recipe I appropriated from Cesare that I love. You chop up rosemary, garlic, and parsley and stuff it in the cavity, then douse the fish with lemon juice and wine as it cooks. It comes out great every time. Jodie says she stir-fries the spring greens, which you can do while the trout is in the oven. Reheat the rice in the microwave, and you're done. It's so simple. While you're at it, make an extra fish, and the next night serve it filleted on top of salad leaves.

As I said before, I am not a high-flying gourmet. You don't have to be one either to put a decent meal on the table. Forget about being intimidated. It's like everything else. If you're not good at something, practise. As you get better at it, you will enjoy it more. And while you're enjoying cooking more, you'll eat better and eat out less. You'll also get thinner, because you will be at home and have more control over portion size. I promise. It doesn't have to be trout with spring greens and rice, if that's not your thing. Start with more familiar dishes and foods you can prepare in advance and just reheat.

That is why there are women's magazines. You know the ones, suggesting strategies for meals that last for a week, or making a pot of black beans that start off as a salad, then slip into burrito mode, then finish as beans and rice or tostadas. There are chicken breasts that turn into fajitas, chicken parmesan, and tortilla soup. A meat sauce with rump steaks can go over pasta one night; add chunks of carrots, potatoes, and beans later in the week, and you've got a hearty stew.

The main thing is, you don't have to try very hard. All you really need is a few simple ingredients. Maybe fajitas and tortilla soup are more than you want to tackle. In that case, strip it down. Manhattanites get ribbed for their obsession with fancy stuff like scallops, extra-virgin olive oil, and gourmet mushrooms. But you can't beat top-quality ingredients. If you start with the right building blocks, the food will do the work for you.

Trend watchers like to point to the shrinking number of items in a meal as a sign of the decline of interest in cooking. Back in the 1980s, the average number of items in a meal was 4.4; in 2010, it was 3.5, according to NPD, a market research firm. The explanation given is convenience, and I am sure that's right. Yet I repeat, you don't need a hundred ingredients to make a fantastic meal. In summer, buy tomatoes in season, slice them on a plate with some buffalo mozzarella and fresh basil, and drizzle with extra-virgin olive oil, and you will have a Caprese salad, a perfect dish. Perfect. No cooking at all. Or throw together a modified Niçoise salad, with great tuna (in olive oil, not water—it tastes much better), salad leaves, olives, anchovies, and, if you're feeling ambitious, boiled green beans. Add a small slice of crusty bread, and you're done.

I've actually streamlined my cooking significantly over the years. I remember that when I first came to New York, I used to make an elaborate ratatouille that involved salting and draining aubergine, peeling tomatoes, and pitting olives. I made spanakopita, a Greek spinach pie that called for cooking down pounds of fresh spinach and mint and buttering paper-thin layers of filo pastry. That's fine, if you have the time, but who needs it? Cesare has taught me to keep things simple. It's the whole foundation of the Italian kitchen.

My mother-in-law enjoys a dish of sautéed Swiss chard and a slice of grilled bread rubbed with garlic and oil and calls it dinner. And honestly, with good olive oil, garlic, kosher salt, and pepper, you can make a delicious meal of almost anything. When I came home from work one day, Cesare surprised me with some roasted branzino, a white-flesh fish. It sounds complicated, but all he did was pour on a little oil, sprinkle it with salt and pepper, put slices of tomato and lettuce on top, and pop it in the oven. A meal like that is one of the many lovely things about being married to Cesare, and it was heavenly. I've made it myself many times since.

Conclusion: there is no need for a frozen low-fat dinner or a salad made with zero-calorie dressing. You can make it yourself for less, it will taste better, and you'll spend just a little more time on it. If you get good at it, you can whip up a tasty meal in almost the time it takes to microwave. I keep staples on hand all the time—I make steamed brown rice every few days and a pot of chickpeas or another legume once a week. (For when I forget to soak the beans, I keep a few cans on hand, too.) Then I let loose in the vegetable department. I buy whatever is fresh and sauté or roast the vegetables with garlic and dried chilli flakes.

It almost echoes those diets that keep you eating one thing—a baked potato, cabbage soup, grapefruit, or whatever—except that the foods aren't theoretically dietetic, they're de facto dietetic. They're good whole foods that fill you up. They satisfy you emotionally and physically, so you don't find yourself fishing around in the fridge at 10 p.m. because you're still hungry or because you want to reward yourself for having a 400-calorie frozen dinner.

Also, you're not running a restaurant. You don't need Eric Ripert's repertoire to eat well. Joanna Coles, the editor of *Marie Claire*, remembers that when she was a child, her mom made the same dishes every week. On Sunday it was a roast, on Monday it was cold meats. On Tuesday, chops; on Wednesday, fish and chips. In that generation, I think it was a pretty common approach. My mom wasn't quite so rigid, but she had about six or seven things she knew how to do well and rotated them—things like baked chicken, macaroni and cheese, and hamburgers. Now, because of the Food Network and other stations' cooking shows, women think they have to be like a professional chef and prepare a multicourse international extravaganza night after night. Not true! Figure out four or five things you love that are easy for you to prepare, and stick with them. When you're in the mood, you can retire whatever is boring you and add something new.

. . . .

The Amateurs Weigh In

Best Dinners in Less than Half an Hour

Scrambled eggs with spinach

Store-roasted chicken with greens and precooked brown rice

Wholewheat pasta with an anchovy paste sauce, topped with breadcrumbs and parsley.

Pasta puttanesca

Green salad with roasted Brussels sprouts, red pepper, cheese, sugar snap peas, and turkey chunks

Pasta with sausage and broccoli or asparagus, fresh green beans, and courgettes

Grilled salmon with bruschetta salsa and green beans

Salad leaves, warm butter beans, red onion, garlic, olive oil, wine vinegar, and tuna

Pasta with mussels

Cookbooks I Can't Live Without

Deborah Madison's Vegetarian Cooking for Everyone by Deborah Madison

Joy of Cooking by Irma Rombauer

Lulu Powers Food to Flowers by Lulu Powers

The Silver Palate Cookbook by Julee Rosso and Sheila Lukins

America's Test Kitchen Family Cookbook by America's Test Kitchen

Gourmet Cookbook by *Gourmet* editors

How to Cook Everything by Mark Bittman

The Classic Italian Cookbook by Marcella Hazan

Yan Can Cook by Martin Yang

Lidia's Family Table by Lidia Bastianich

. . . .

One fail-proof place to start is with a baking tray and some vegetables—the ones the government keeps telling us to eat more of. I roast cauliflower, broccoli, carrots, sweet potatoes, kale, green beans, parsnips, acorn squash, radicchio, butternut squash, corn, edamame, and tomatoes, to name a few. Sometimes I do combos: root vegetables are especially good together. Sometimes it's just a vegetable solo. Either way, just sprinkle with olive oil, salt, and dried chilli flakes. Make enough for two or three nights and reheat.

I'm not saying everyone has to cook this way, but you can't go wrong sticking to the basic concept. Keep it simple, keep it quality. "Every meal doesn't have to be perfect," says Shaw, the

International Culinary Center instructor. "If you make what's filling and satisfying, you don't need a box of biscuits."

A word of warning: this approach isn't going to be cheap. Imported tuna in olive oil will cost $12 (£7.50) or so for 225 grams, about seven times as much as a supermarket brand in vegetable oil. Buffalo mozzarella, to make the Caprese salad described earlier, will cost about 40 percent more than the ordinary kind. You can pay $9 (£5.50) or $3.50 (£2) for anchovies. But you won't be sorry if you spend the extra money. The food will taste so much better, and you won't have to put so much work into dinner.

You might even help reverse the trend Pew found in 2006 when it asked adults if they enjoy eating "a great deal" and found that only 39 percent said yes, which was down from 48 percent in 1989. What a disheartening statistic. No wonder people keep getting fatter. They don't taste the food they eat, and in all likelihood they don't even feel as though they've eaten anything.

I don't mean to sound like a shill for the olive oil council, but the place to start is with the best extra-virgin olive oil you can afford. I say this for two reasons. First, many dieters (myself included) are too afraid of fat. Olive oil is good for your skin, good for your digestion, and good for your health. The good fats and in the right amounts will not make you gain weight. So put your irrational fears aside and buy some—and use it.

Second, extra-virgin olive oil will make all of your food taste better with no effort at all. You will notice right away. My favourite is called Laudemio. It's made by an aristocratic Italian family, the Frescobaldis, who also produce some fantastic wines—and they charge dearly for both. The olive oil is $42 (£26) for just under 500 millilitres at Dean & DeLuca. I use it on salads and as a condiment, like salt and pepper, to flavor soups, pastas, and meats. For actual cooking—sautéing, in sauces, and so on—I buy a lesser quality, usually the Fairway house brand, but Colavita, or even the Costco house brand is fine. Think of it this way: how much have you spent in your life on diets? What's another $40 (£25) once or twice a year for a bottle of oil you use sparingly, especially if it actually works?

I know you know what I'm about to say; you've read it in magazines and heard about it on television. Yet tomorrow you're going to look up a recipe for 500 grams of Brussels sprouts, green beans, or roasted corn, and it's going to call for half a teaspoon of olive oil and a non-stick pan or some such nonsense. Discard those instructions. They're ridiculous. You will not only ruin perfectly good ingredients, you will burn the pan. Use a tablespoon or two. You don't need half a bottle. Theresa Passarelli tells me she goes through about two and a half litres of olive oil a month. I'm probably in the same neighbourhood. As I was watching Myriam make her omelette, I noted she had at least 50 millilitres of oil in the pan. Good fat makes you feel full! That's how it makes or keeps you slim. You get the idea.

I understand there are plenty of good reasons people don't cook. They think they don't do it very well. They don't have the time or the patience. I recently read that the percentage of women who enjoy cooking a meal keeps declining. When researchers asked women about cooking back in 1989, 39 percent said they enjoyed making a meal. But when asked the same question in 2006, only 35 percent were still keen on it. This is a shame. And like the fact that people are enjoying eating less, it is so telling about Americans in general. We like cooking less and eating less than we used to, yet we are fatter than we've ever been.

I can't believe there isn't a connection here. The human body is so sophisticated. It has needs we can't process intellectually. We demonize carbs, yet they are crucial for brain and muscle function. We eat fat-free yogurt, even though we need fat for cell growth, to produce hormones, and to absorb certain nutrients. We are worried about a number on the scale while our bodies are scrambling to find the specific fuels they need to operate. We are eating and preparing really awful food. We've replaced quality with quantity. No wonder our bodies are fatter than ever. They're in rebellion. The body is seeking a protein-rich filet mignon, a few perfectly roasted seasonal vegetables, and a cup of barley, but instead we're eating multiple servings of Lean Cuisine.

At least, that's what I think. It's time to change it. Fire up your stove and make a delicious dinner.

Manhattan Diet Secrets

- *Cooking will help you to maintain a healthy weight*. It gives you control over the ingredients, the way the food is cooked, and how it tastes. It's also emotionally satisfying. You will be more connected to your meal. This really works. If you don't believe me, talk to the French.

- *Olive oil is good for you*. This is crucial. Lots of people have written about the trap of low-fat diets. Low-fat makes you fat! It's true. Why have Americans gotten progressively bigger with the proliferation of spa cuisine, low-fat crackers, and fat-free yogurt? It's too much to go into right here, but many studies have shown that olive oil is good for you. You don't even have to read them. Just look at the Italians. Olive oil tastes good. It's healthy. Dump the oil spray. Buy a bottle of extra-virgin olive oil.

- *Want to become a great cook fast?* Buy really good ingredients. It's almost that easy. Better food means you're eating better. Just remember portion control.

- *Keep it simple*. You don't have to labour over duck flambé. The more straightforward the recipe, the better. The less time spent shopping and the less time spent cooking, the easier it is to pull off. Fresh herbs like rosemary, thyme, and sage can transform a boring pork chop into a Tuscan feast. The other night I made pasta with chunks of mozzarella and mortadella. It was simple and delicious.

- *Roast, roast, roast.* It takes about twenty minutes to roast most vegetables. Broccoli and cauliflower get brown and crispy. If you use sweet potato or butternut squash in a root vegetable mix, the vegetables caramelize for a honey-like flavor. Kale gets super flaky and breaks up almost like crisps—but with beta-carotene, vitamin A, and no saturated fat.

11

A Spoonful at a Time
The Manhattan Diet Recipes

BREAKFAST
Lauren Lipton's Porridge
Sarah Powers's Spinach Scramble
Courgette Frittata
Pam Liebman's Egg White and
  Oat Waffles
Oat and Egg White Pancakes
Bread and Courage Golden
  Granola

SANDWICHES AND SOUPS
Greek Salad Pitta
Christine Baranski's Butternut
  Squash Soup

Carrot Soup
Lentil Soup
Mushroom Soup

PASTA
Pasta with Sautéed Broccoli
Orzo with Spinach
Wholewheat Linguine with
  Roasted Cauliflower
Pasta with Black Olives
Pasta with Salmon and Asparagus
Wholewheat Pasta with Anchovy
  Sauce
Red Wine Risotto

MEAT, FISH, AND POULTRY

Turkey Tacos

Joanna Coles's Shepherd's Pie

Prawns and Beans

Turkey Chilli

Turkey Meatballs

Plaice Fillets on Parchment

Tandoori Salmon

Prawn Tortillas

Chicken Milanese

Tofu Stir-Fry

Black-Eyed Beans with Bacon and Bitter Greens

Rosemary Pork Chops

Cristina Cuomo's Roasted Chicken with Root Vegetables

Rosemary-Roasted Trout

Tom Colicchio's Poached Sea Bass with Roasted Tomato Vinaigrette and Fennel Salad

Eric Ripert's Grilled Salmon and Herb Salad with Toasted Sesame Seeds and Ponzu Vinaigrette

Lidia Bastianich's Pan-Fried Chicken Breasts *Aglio e Olio*

Mussels in Sake

SIDE DISHES, SALADS, AND VEGETABLES

Chopped Salad Niçoise

Rocket and Chestnut Mushroom Salad

Sautéed Spinach (or Swiss Chard)

Asparagus Salad

Spring Greens in Spicy Tomato Sauce

Black Bean, Sweetcorn, and Tomato Salad

Chicken Salad with Radicchio and Pine Nuts

Roasted Radicchio

Tuscan Tuna Salad

Chicken Salad

Salmon Salad

Roasted Root Vegetables

Roasted Butternut Squash

Tomato Bruschetta

Bruschetta with Beans

Caesar Salad

Marcus Samuelsson's Tomato-Watermelon Salad with Almond Vinaigrette

Lentil Salad

Avocado and Grapefruit Salad with Citrus Dressing

Spinach Salad with Artichokes and Lemon Dressing

Roasted Kale Crisps

Mario Batali's Misticanza

SALAD DRESSINGS, DIPS, AND SPREADS

Asian-Style Dressing for Green Beans or Salad Greens

Vinaigrette

Honey-Dijon Dressing

Erika's Olive Tapenade

Lemony Hummus

Spinach Dip

Anchovy Dip

DESSERTS

Chocolate Pudding

Chocolate Peanut Butter Pudding

Oat Cookies

I collected recipes from my journal keepers and from New York chefs. I also adapted a dozen or so from recipes that Cesare has taught me over the years, other dishes we make at home, and a few from a cookbook we did together years ago, *Diary of a Tuscan Chef*. In adapting the recipes, I typically cut down on the oil and increased the amount of vegetables.

BREAKFAST

Lauren Lipton's Porridge

SERVES 1

My friend Lauren the novelist has this for breakfast almost every morning and maintains it's the key to her slimness. It's easy to prepare and full of fibre and calcium. I would prepare it with whole milk and make stove-top porridge, but I don't want to mess with her recipe.

- 30g instant porridge oats
- 300ml semi-skimmed milk
- 40g raisins
- 2 tablespoons sliced almonds
- 2 tablespoons ground flaxseeds
- 1 small apple, diced
- 1 tablespoon honey

Mix all the ingredients together in a medium-size bowl and prepare the porridge in the microwave according to the packet instructions.

. . . .

Sarah Powers's Spinach Scramble

SERVES 1

Sarah works in the wine and spirits industry and eats out five or six nights a week. When she's home, she keeps it simple with things like this egg and spinach dish. You can also add pesto and/or parmesan cheese to these eggs for a richer flavour.

olive oil spray

1 whole egg, plus 3 egg whites

splash of water

30g chopped fresh spinach (or 80g cooked chopped frozen spinach)

salt and freshly ground black pepper to taste

1–2 tablespoons pesto sauce (optional)

1 tablespoon parmesan cheese (optional)

Spray a pan with the olive oil and heat to medium-high. Whisk the eggs together with the water. When the pan is hot, add the eggs, lower the heat to low-medium, and stir. When the eggs have started to solidify with not much liquid left, add the spinach and salt and pepper. (If desired, add pesto sauce and/or parmesan cheese at this point.) Stir it all together. Allow to set briefly, then serve.

. . . .

Courgette Frittata

SERVES 4

This is a light variation on scarpaccia, a dish Cesare makes for us sometimes on Sunday mornings or when we are weekend guests at friends' country homes.

1 tablespoon extra-virgin olive oil

1 tablespoon finely chopped garlic

1 tablespoon chopped oregano

1 tablespoon chopped thyme

½ teaspoon dried chilli flakes

250g thinly sliced red onion

450g thinly sliced courgette

1 whole egg plus 2 egg whites

4 tablespoons flour

4 tablespoons water

4 tablespoons chopped flat-leaf parsley

salt and freshly ground black pepper

1 tablespoon parmesan cheese

1 tablespoon pecorino-romano cheese

olive oil spray

Preheat the oven to 200°C/gas mark 6.

In a medium non-stick frying pan, heat the oil, garlic, oregano, thyme, and chilli flakes over a medium flame for about 3 minutes. Add the onions and continue sautéing, stirring occasionally, for 5 minutes. Add the courgettes and cook for another 7–10 minutes, stirring occasionally until the onions and courgettes are almost translucent. Remove the pan from the heat and cool.

In a bowl, beat together the eggs, flour, water, parsley, salt and pepper, and cheeses. Mix in the courgettes and onions.

Spray two 10-inch cake tins with the oil and heat in the oven for a few minutes. Remove the tins and pour half of the courgette mixture into each. Bake for 15–20 minutes.

. . . .

Pam Liebman's Egg White and Oat Waffles

SERVES 1

Pam runs one of the largest residential property businesses in New York City and stays in incredible shape. I would take her diet advice on anything.

125g egg whites (about 4)

40g organic oats (not instant)

60ml water

dash cinnamon

fresh berries

syrup or jam (optional)

Mix the egg whites, oats, water, and cinnamon in a blender. Pour the mixture into a waffle iron and cook.

Serve with fresh berries on top. Add syrup or jam, if you like.

Variation
For a different, lighter flavour, add the following to the egg white, oat, and water mixture: 50g low-fat cottage cheese and 1 teaspoon lemon juice.

. . . .

Oat and Egg White Pancakes
SERVES 1

Inspired by Pam's waffle recipe, I made pancakes. Remarkably, they resemble testaroli, a pancake-like pasta from the tiny Tuscan town of Pontremoli. Testaroli are served with pesto, and a dab of that on these pancakes is fantastic.

125g egg whites (about 4)
40g old-fashioned rolled oats
1 tablespoon water
salt

Put the egg whites, rolled oats, water, and salt in a blender and puree. Heat a non-stick 8-inch frying pan over a medium flame. Pour in half of the batter and cook about 45 seconds on each side. Repeat and serve.

. . . .

Bread and Courage Golden Granola
SERVES 8

This granola is incredibly rich (butter will do that) and satisfying. A little bit goes a long way. I will have a small amount as a dessert. Christine Baranksi, who passed the recipe on, has it as a late-night snack. The recipe is from her daughter Isabel Cowles, who writes about food on her blog, Bread and Courage.

225g butter

250g local honey

350g old-fashioned rolled oats

75g coarsely chopped walnuts

75g coarsely chopped almonds

75g coarsely chopped cashews

75g sunflower seeds

1 teaspoon salt

35g shredded coconut

150g dried fruit (cranberries are my favorite for this)

Preheat the oven to 160°C/gas mark 3.

Place the butter and honey in a saucepan over a low heat and stir until the butter melts.

Put the oats, walnuts, almonds, cashews, and sunflower seeds in a large bowl. Coat with half of the hot butter mixture and stir to combine. Spread evenly over a non-stick or parchment-paper-lined baking sheet.

Bake for 10 minutes, then remove from the oven. Add the remaining butter mixture, then sprinkle the salt all over.

Sprinkle the coconut flakes on top—these help to absorb any butter that is not being picked up by the oats. Stir again, if necessary.

Bake another 5 minutes, then stir a final time, being sure that the coconut and oats are evenly redistributed. Add the fruit and bake an additional 5 minutes.

Cool, then store in an airtight container.

SANDWICHES AND SOUPS

Greek Salad Pitta

SERVES 1

I love Greek salad. It's refreshing, filling, and healthy.

1 wholemeal pitta

25g feta, crumbled

100g chopped tomato

50g chopped cucumber

40g chopped green pepper

4 black olives, chopped

¼ teaspoon dried oregano

1 teaspoon extra-virgin olive oil

1–2 teaspoons red wine vinegar

salt and freshly ground black pepper

Slice the edge off the pitta to open. In a bowl, mix the feta, tomato, cucumber, pepper, and olives. Sprinkle with oregano and add the olive oil, then add the vinegar, and toss. Add salt and pepper to taste. Stuff the mixture into the pitta and serve.

. . . .

Christine Baranski's Butternut Squash Soup

SERVES 6

Christine got this recipe from her daughter, Isabel Cowles, who adapted it from Gourmet *for her blog,* Bread and Courage. *It's Christine's favourite soup to serve guests.*

2 tablespoons olive oil

150g diced onion

1 teaspoon finely chopped garlic

1 x 400g can whole tomatoes, chopped, reserve liquid

550g butternut squash, cut into 1-cm cubes

1–2 tablespoons chopped fresh sage (and some extra for garnish)

1 litre vegetable (or chicken) stock

salt and freshly ground black pepper

1 x 400g can cannellini beans, drained and rinsed

toasted pumpkin seeds (for garnish)

parmesan cheese (for garnish)

Heat the olive oil in a large, heavy-bottomed soup pot. Add the onions and cook over a medium flame for 10–15 minutes, until they are translucent. Add the garlic and cook about 4 minutes, until slightly brown.

Deglaze the pot with tomato juice from the can of tomatoes and then add the tomatoes, squash, sage, and stock. Add salt and pepper to taste.

Bring the soup to the boil, then turn down the heat and simmer for 30 minutes or until the squash is soft and the stock has reduced somewhat.

To thicken the soup, smash the cubes of squash against the sides of the pot.

At this point, the soup can be refrigerated for up to three days. Reheat the soup and add the beans about 15 minutes before serving.

Garnish with the extra sage and toasted pumpkin seeds or parmesan.

. . . .

Carrot Soup

SERVES 4

This recipe comes to me from an old colleague, Julie Belcove, who got it from her roommate at Harvard.

1 tablespoon olive oil

80g chopped onion

350g peeled, sliced carrots

100g peeled, diced potatoes

50g sliced celery

750ml chicken stock

225ml milk or 1 tablespoon Greek yogurt (optional)

¼ teaspoon salt

⅛ teaspoon freshly ground black pepper

Heat the olive oil in a large soup pot. Add the onions and sauté over a medium flame for about 7 minutes, until they are translucent. Add the other vegetables and the chicken stock and stir. Cover and simmer about 20 minutes, until tender.

Remove the soup from the heat and puree in batches. You can make this as smooth or as chunky as you like.

Return to the heat and add the milk or yogurt, if you are using it, and salt and pepper.

. . . .

Lentil Soup

SERVES 8

The mustard is the secret ingredient in this soup.

1 tablespoon olive oil

150g chopped onion

125g chopped carrot

100g chopped celery

1 tablespoon chopped garlic

4 sprigs fresh sage or 1 teaspoon dried sage

500ml red or white wine

1 x 400g can Italian tomatoes

250g dried green lentils, rinsed and picked through to remove stones

2 litres water

2–3 tablespoons Dijon mustard

2 tablespoons tomato paste

salt and freshly ground pepper

Heat the oil in a large saucepan and sauté the onions, carrots, celery, garlic, and sage over a medium flame until the onions begin to brown. Add the wine and cook until it evaporates completely.

Crush the tomatoes with your hands and add to the pot. Cook 5 minutes, then add the lentils and water. Bring the mixture to the boil, reduce the heat, and simmer for 20 minutes. Test the lentils to see whether they're cooked. They should be tender.

Stir in the mustard and tomato paste and add the salt and pepper to taste. If you like a creamy soup, put half of the mixture into a food processor and pulse, then return the puree to the pot and cook another 5 minutes.

. . . .

Mushroom Soup

SERVES 4

1 x 75g pack dried porcini mushrooms

125ml boiling water

5 teaspoons olive oil

200g diced onion

75g diced carrot

50g diced celery

2 teaspoons finely chopped garlic

1 tablespoon chopped fresh rosemary

500g chestnut mushrooms, cleaned and chopped

1 litre vegetable stock

2 tablespoons tomato puree

salt and freshly ground black pepper

Place the porcini mushrooms in a small bowl and cover with the boiling water. Leave to soak for 30 minutes.

In a large pot, stir together the oil, onion, carrot, celery, garlic, and rosemary. Sauté over a medium flame for about 15 minutes, until the vegetables are soft.

Gently remove the porcini from their soaking liquid. Reserve the liquid. Chop the porcini and add to the vegetable mixture along with the chestnut mushrooms. Sauté for 5 minutes more.

Pour the vegetable stock into the pot, add the tomato puree, and stir. Season with the salt and pepper and simmer for 25 minutes. Line a sieve with a paper towel. Hold the sieve over the soup and pour in the liquid from the mushrooms. Simmer another 5 minutes and serve.

. . . .

PASTA

Pasta with Sautéed Broccoli

SERVES 2

After salad and baby carrots, broccoli was the single most popular vegetable with my dieters. You can eat it alone, with pasta, as in this recipe, or on top of a piece of crusty toast.

1 teaspoon salt, plus 1 tablespoon
200g broccoli, with ends trimmed
125g short pasta, such as bowties or orecchiette
1 tablespoon olive oil
2 teaspoons finely chopped garlic
½ teaspoon dried chilli flakes
salt and freshly ground black pepper

Fill a large pot with 2 inches of water. Add the teaspoon of salt and bring it to a low boil. Add the broccoli and cover, steaming for 7–8 minutes. Drain in a colander and cool. When the broccoli is cool enough to handle, chop roughly and set aside.

In a medium pot, bring a litre of water to the boil and add the tablespoon of salt and the pasta of your choice. Cook 10 minutes or until al dente.

Meanwhile, in a non-stick frying pan, heat the oil, garlic, and chilli flakes over a medium flame until the garlic turns golden. Add the broccoli and stir until the flavours are mixed. Add the salt and pepper to taste. Mix with the pasta and serve.

. . . .

Orzo with Spinach

SERVES 2

I started making this instead of risotto because the orzo, which is a type of pasta, cooks twice as fast as Arborio rice. You also don't have to stand over the stove stirring as you do with risotto, so it's easier on the cook. Even my mother-in-law, Rosa, likes it, which is a very big compliment.

1 tablespoon olive oil
150g chopped red onion
½ teaspoon dried chilli flakes
100g orzo
½–1 litre simmering chicken stock
2 tablespoons tomato paste
275g frozen chopped spinach, thawed
1 tablespoon grated parmesan cheese
1 tablespoon grated pecorino-romano cheese

Place the oil, onion, and chilli flakes in a medium saucepan. Sauté over a medium flame for about 10 minutes, until the onions are caramelized. Stir in the orzo and mix well. Let it toast for 1–2 minutes, then add 500ml of the simmering chicken stock. Stir, then add the tomato paste and spinach. Simmer for 9–10 minutes, adding more stock if the mixture gets dry. Stir in the cheeses and serve.

. . . .

Wholewheat Linguine with Roasted Cauliflower

SERVES 2

300g cauliflower florets, rinsed, with water clinging to the
florets

1 clove garlic

1 tablespoon olive oil

2 teaspoons salt, plus 1 tablespoon

1 teaspoon dried chilli flakes

225g wholewheat linguine (or other pasta)

1 tablespoon chopped flat-leaf parsley

salt and freshly ground pepper

2 tablespoons grated parmesan cheese

Preheat the oven to 220°C/gas mark 7.

Place the cauliflower and garlic clove in a bowl and toss
with the olive oil, the 2 teaspoons of salt, and the chilli flakes.
Place on a baking sheet and roast in the oven for 10 minutes.
Stir and roast for another 10 minutes. Remove when the florets are toasted at the edges.

While the cauliflower is cooking, fill a medium pot with
water and the tablespoon of salt. Bring to the boil and add the
pasta. Cook for 10 minutes or until al dente. Drain, reserving
125ml cooking liquid.

In a serving bowl, mix the cauliflower and pasta together,
adding the parsley, salt, and pepper. If the pasta seems a little
dry, add some of the reserved cooking liquid. Sprinkle with
the parmesan cheese and serve.

. . . .

Pasta with Black Olives

SERVES 2

This is one of the easiest dinners I know.

125g short pasta, such as fusilli

1 tablespoon salt

100g black olives (You can pit and chop them or leave whole. I prefer them whole—more to chew.)

2 teaspoons olive oil

½ teaspoon dried chilli flakes

2 teaspoons finely chopped flat-leaf parsley

salt and freshly ground black pepper

In a medium pot, bring a litre of water to the boil and add the pasta and salt. Cook for 10 minutes or until al dente. Drain and toss well with the remaining ingredients. Serve.

. . . .

Pasta with Salmon and Asparagus

SERVES 2

Cesare and I included a more robust version of this recipe in Diary of a Tuscan Chef. *I adapted it here so there are more vegetables and less oil.*

1 tablespoon olive oil

2 teaspoons finely chopped garlic

½ teaspoon dried chilli flakes

1 sprig fresh rosemary

225g asparagus, cut into 1-inch lengths, tips set aside

1 tablespoon finely chopped flat-leaf parsley

125g salmon fillet, thinly sliced

1 medium tomato, peeled and chopped

salt and freshly ground black pepper

225g short pasta, such as fusilli, penne, or bowties

Place the olive oil, garlic, red pepper, rosemary, and asparagus (not the tips) in a non-stick frying pan and sauté over a medium-high flame for about 5 minutes or until the garlic starts to colour and the asparagus is bright green. Add the parsley and stir. Add the salmon and cook for 2–3 minutes.

Add the tomato, salt, pepper, and asparagus tips. Lower the heat and cook another 2 minutes. Set aside but keep warm.

Bring a medium-sized pot of salted water to the boil. Add the pasta and cook for about 8 minutes, until it is very al dente. Drain and add the pasta to the salmon mixture. Cook another 2–3 minutes and serve.

. . . .

Wholewheat Pasta with Anchovy Sauce
SERVES 2

I have cut the olive oil down in this recipe, which is an Italian favourite.

100g short, wholewheat pasta
1 tablespoon salt
2 tablespoons olive oil
2 cloves garlic, sliced
¼ teaspoon dried chilli flakes
5–10 anchovies, rinsed and chopped
1 tablespoon finely chopped flat-leaf parsley
40g plain breadcrumbs

In a medium pot, bring a litre of water to the boil and add the pasta and salt. Cook for about 8 minutes, until very al dente. Drain, reserving 125ml cooking liquid.

While the pasta is cooking, heat the olive oil in a large non-stick frying pan. Add the garlic slices and sauté over a medium-low flame until the garlic is golden brown. Remove the garlic and discard or save for another dish. Add the chilli flakes and the chopped anchovies and continue cooking, stirring occasionally, until the anchovies dissolve. Turn off the heat, add the pasta to the pan, along with a little of the cooking water, and heat another minute. Toss with the parsley. Top with the breadcrumbs and serve.

. . . .

Red Wine Risotto

SERVES 2

Traditional risotto recipes call for the laborious ladling of the liquid, 100ml at a time, and lots of butter. I don't think either are necessary. Add the liquid all at once and no one will be the wiser, but you do need to keep stirring.

> 1 tablespoon olive oil
> 75g chopped red onion
> 150g Arborio rice
> 150ml chicken stock
> 125ml red wine
> salt and pepper to taste
> 2 tablespoons grated parmesan cheese

Place the olive oil and onion in a medium saucepan and heat over a medium flame until the onion is translucent, about 10 minutes. Add the rice and toast it, stirring constantly for 1–2 minutes.

While the rice is toasting, in a small saucepan bring the chicken stock and wine to a low simmer. Add all of the liquid to the rice and reduce the heat to a low simmer. Add the salt and pepper. Cook, stirring constantly, for about 15–18 minutes. When the rice is done, it should be al dente, or firm to the bite. Stir in the grated parmesan cheese and serve immediately.

MEAT, FISH, AND POULTRY
Turkey Tacos

SERVES 4, TWO TACOS APIECE

One of the biggest surprises for me was to see how many Manhattanites cook with turkey mince instead of finely chopped beef. I

spoon mine over salad and top it with chopped tomatoes and a
scant tablespoon of grated cheddar.

1 tablespoon olive oil

1 tablespoon finely chopped garlic

75g chopped onion

2 jalapeños, seeds removed, finely chopped

1 teaspoon cumin (more or less to taste)

1 teaspoon chilli powder

1 teaspoon dried oregano

600g turkey mince

3 tablespoons lime juice

4 tablespoons finely chopped coriander

8 hard taco shells, warmed briefly (or use lettuce leaves)

200g chopped tomato (for garnish)

50g chopped lettuce (for garnish)

4 tablespoons grated cheddar (optional)

In a large non-stick frying pan, heat the oil and sauté the garlic, onion, and jalapeños until soft. Add the cumin, chilli powder, and oregano and stir. Add the turkey mince, breaking it up into small chunks. When the meat is completely cooked through, turn off the heat and stir in the lime juice and coriander.

Spoon the meat into the taco shells (or on top of a bed of lettuce). Garnish with tomato and lettuce and grated cheddar, if desired.

. . . .

Joanna Coles's Shepherd's Pie
SERVES 8

Joanna's mom made this for her when she was growing up in England. She likes it with peas or green beans and says it is easily reheatable and good for entertaining. You can make it a day before or make the meat sauce in big batches and freeze it. I reduced the amount of olive oil.

1½ tablespoons olive oil, plus 1 tablespoon

2 teaspoons finely chopped garlic

400g chopped onions

3 tablespoons red wine

1.5kg organic mince beef

2 x 400g cans chopped tomatoes

1 x 142g can tomato paste

1 tablespoon Worcestershire sauce

1.5kg potatoes, peeled and quartered

1 tablespoon butter

60ml milk, as needed

60g grated mature cheddar cheese

Preheat the oven to 180°C/gas mark 4.

Heat the 1½ tablespoons of oil in a heavy-bottomed frying pan and sauté the garlic and onions over a medium flame for about 10 minutes, until they are translucent. Add the red wine and stir until it evaporates. Add the mince and brown thoroughly. Stir in the chopped tomatoes, tomato paste, and Worcestershire sauce. Cook until there is no liquid left in the pan. Set aside.

Bring a large pot of salted water to the boil and add the potatoes. Cook for about 20 minutes, until tender. Drain. Mash by hand or in a blender with the remaining 1 tablespoon of oil, the butter, and the milk as needed.

Put the meat sauce in an ovenproof serving dish, layer the mashed potatoes on top of it, and sprinkled the grated cheese over the potatoes. Bake for 30 minutes. Turn the oven to grill and heat the cheese for 3 minutes to brown the top.

. . . .

Prawns and Beans

SERVES 2

Cesare's friend Romano in Viareggio, Italy, makes the best prawns and beans I've ever had. The key is exquisite prawns, good-quality beans, and fancy extra-virgin olive oil. Buy the best you can find.

225g raw prawns

60ml cider vinegar

ice bath

75g cooked cannellini beans, drained and rinsed

100g chopped tomato

2 tablespoons chopped fresh basil

2 teaspoons extra-virgin olive oil

2 teaspoons red wine vinegar

salt and freshly ground black pepper

1 head Little Gem lettuce, cleaned and torn into bite-size pieces

Place the prawns in a saucepan and cover with 2 inches of salted water. Add the cider vinegar. Heat the water to just under a simmer. Don't let it boil, and stir the prawns constantly. When one or two prawns float to the surface, turn off the heat, drain immediately, and dump the prawns into the ice bath to stop the cooking process. Drain well.

In a bowl, combine the prawns, beans, tomato, and basil. Season with the olive oil, red wine vinegar, salt, and pepper.

Divide the lettuce onto two plates. Spoon half the prawn mixture onto each plate and serve.

. . . .

Turkey Chilli

SERVES 8

The author of this recipe, my friend Janet Ungless, is one of the healthiest eaters I know. Ergo, this recipe is fail-proof.

olive oil spray

1 tablespoon finely chopped garlic

150g chopped onion

500g turkey mince

1 x 400g can whole peeled tomatoes

1 x 400g can kidney beans, drained and rinsed

2 teaspoons coriander

2 teaspoons cumin

2 tablespoons chilli powder

2 teaspoons dried oregano

salt and freshly ground black pepper

½ teaspoon cayenne pepper

Spray a non-stick frying pan with olive oil, heat over a medium flame, and sauté the garlic and onions for about 10 minutes, until the onions are translucent. Add the turkey mince and continue cooking, breaking up the meat with a wooden spoon.

In a medium-size bowl, crush the whole tomatoes with your hands. Add the tomatoes and their juice to the turkey mixture. Add the remaining ingredients and simmer for 10–15 minutes. Serve.

. . . .

Turkey Meatballs

MAKES 20 MEATBALLS

Turkey meatballs are a family-friendly recipe. My friend Hilary serves them on top of spaghetti to her kids and with a green vegetable, like sautéed Swiss chard or broccoli, for herself. You can also use the meatballs in sandwiches.

2 tablespoons olive oil

400g chopped onion, plus 75g finely finely chopped

1 tablespoon finely chopped garlic, plus 2 teaspoons

1 teaspoon fresh or dried oregano

salt and freshly ground black pepper

150g carrot, peeled and chopped

1 x 400g can plum tomatoes

500g turkey mince

Heat 1 tablespoon of the oil in a frying pan and sauté the 400g onion and the 1 tablespoon garlic over a medium flame for about 5 minutes, until the vegetables are soft and fragrant. Add the oregano, salt and pepper, and carrots. Continue cooking for about 5 more minutes, until the carrots are tender. Break up the tomatoes into chunks and add to the frying pan. Leave the sauce to simmer while you prepare the meatballs.

In a large bowl, combine the turkey with the 75g onion, the 2 teaspoons garlic, and salt and pepper. Form into balls, about the diameter of a 50-pence piece. Heat the remaining tablespoon of oil in a large frying pan. Add the meatballs and sauté over medium until they are browned. You will have to cook them in batches. As the meatballs are done, transfer them to the tomato sauce. They should simmer in the sauce for about 30 minutes. Serve.

. . . .

Plaice Fillets on Parchment

SERVES 4

4 x 125g plaice fillets

2 tablespoons butter

4 teaspoons finely chopped garlic

2 tablespoons chopped flat-leaf parsley or 2 teaspoons dried parsley

salt and freshly ground black pepper

4 lemon wedges

Preheat oven to 200°C/gas mark 6.

Place the fillets on baking parchment. Put 1 teaspoon butter on each piece of fish and sprinkle with 1 teaspoon finely chopped garlic and ½ tablespoon chopped fresh parsley or ½ teaspoon dried parsley. Bake for about 10 minutes.

Sprinkle the fillets with the salt and pepper to taste and serve with a wedge of lemon.

. . . .

Tandoori Salmon

Tandoori without the oven is how I think of this salmon dish. It's from the Family Circle Eat What You Love and Lose *cookbook. I like it with some fragrant basmati rice.*

SERVES 4

Salmon

2 cloves garlic, finely chopped

1 x 1-inch piece fresh ginger, peeled and chopped

1 teaspoon lemon juice

1 teaspoon curry powder

½ teaspoon paprika

½ teaspoon salt

⅛ teaspoon cinnamon

⅛ teaspoon cayenne pepper

700g salmon fillet, 1-inch thick

Raita

125g plain low-fat yogurt

½ cucumber, seeded and thinly sliced

1 teaspoon lemon juice

½ teaspoon salt

Mix the garlic, ginger, lemon juice, and spices. Spread over the salmon. Cover and refrigerate 30 minutes.

Preheat the oven to 230°C/gas mark 8. Bake the salmon 12–15 minutes.

Combine the ingredients for the raita and serve with the salmon.

Prawn Tortillas

SERVES 4

So easy and so good! My friend Hilary, who gave me this recipe, says she also spoons the prawn filling over rice or couscous.

2 tablespoons olive oil

150g chopped onion

1½ tablespoons finely chopped garlic

½ teaspoon dried chilli flakes (or more to taste)

350g cherry tomatoes, halved

salt and freshly ground black pepper

500g prawns, peeled and deveined

4 flour tortillas

Heat the olive oil in a large frying pan and sauté the onions, garlic, and chilli flakes over a medium flame for 4–5 minutes, until fragrant. Add the tomatoes, salt, and pepper. Sauté for about 5 minutes, stirring occasionally. Add the prawns and cook until pink, about 5 minutes, taking care not to overcook.

Warm the tortillas in the microwave. Spoon the prawn mixture into the tortillas and roll them up. Eat them like a sandwich, with your hands, not a fork.

Chicken Milanese

SERVES 2

Use the leftovers in salads or sandwiches or for chicken parmesan.

2 egg whites

2 x 125g chicken breasts

75g seasoned breadcrumbs

1 tablespoon olive oil

salt and freshly ground black pepper

Whisk the egg whites in a small bowl. Dip the cutlets in the whites, then in the breadcrumbs. Heat the olive oil in a medium frying pan. Add the chicken and sauté for 3–4 minutes on each side. Sprinkle with the salt and pepper to taste and serve.

. . . .

Tofu Stir-Fry

SERVES 2

Erika Mansourian was trying to get more veggies into her diet when she came up with this dish. You can substitute almost any vegetable you have at home.

> 400g medium–firm tofu
> 1 tablespoon soy sauce, plus more to taste
> 2 teaspoons sesame oil
> 1 tablespoon rice wine vinegar
> 1½ tablespoons rapeseed oil
> 2 cloves garlic, chopped
> 2 small shallots, diced
> 2 teaspoons fresh ginger, peeled and grated
> 100g button mushrooms, sliced
> 1 medium courgette, sliced
> 1 stalk broccoli, chopped into small florets
> 150g kale, cut into ribbons
> 400g cooked brown rice, kept warm
> 2 tablespoons sesame seeds

Cube the tofu and put it in a bowl with the soy sauce, sesame oil, and rice wine vinegar. Set aside.

Heat the rapeseed oil in a large non-stick frying pan and sauté the garlic and shallots until soft. Add the ginger, the vegetables, and then the tofu. Stir until the vegetables are cooked to your liking. Remove from the heat.

Divide the rice onto two serving plates. Spoon the stir-fry on top and sprinkle the sesame seeds all over. You can also drizzle on some more soy sauce (or tamari) if you like. Serve.

. . . .

Black-Eyed Peas with Bacon and Bitter Greens

SERVES 4

I took this dish from Lauren Lipton, who in turn adapted it from Real Simple *magazine. The original called for endive, but I like even heartier greens like chard, lamb's lettuce and watercress. Sometimes I add a shot of vinegar at the end to brighten the dish. With a little brown rice or other grain, it's a filling dinner.*

4 rashers thick-cut, artisanal bacon

4 cloves garlic, sliced

750g mixed bitter greens—chard, lamb lettuce and water-cress—torn into bite-size pieces

salt and freshly ground black pepper

1 x 400g can black-eyed beans, drained and rinsed

60ml water

1 tablespoon red wine vinegar

Fry the bacon in a large non-stick frying pan over a medium flame for 6–8 minutes, until crisp. Transfer to a plate lined with paper towels.

Add the garlic to the bacon fat and sauté for 1–2 minutes, stirring, until golden brown. Add the greens, season with the salt and pepper, and cook for 2–3 minutes, stirring occasionally, until they begin to wilt.

Add the black-eyed beans and water and simmer 2–3 more minutes. Add the vinegar and toss. Transfer to a serving platter. Chop the bacon into small pieces, sprinkle on top and serve.

. . . .

Rosemary Pork Chops

SERVES 2

Cesare's signature is a sprig of rosemary in his pocket. Just a sprig in this dish perfumes the pork chops.

    2 teaspoons olive oil
    75g chopped shallots
    salt and freshly ground black pepper
    2 x 125g loin chops
    1 sprig rosemary
    60ml white wine

Place the oil and shallots in a large non-stick frying pan and cook over a medium flame for 7–10 minutes, until the shallots are translucent. Season the pork chops with the salt and pepper and add them to the pan, along with the rosemary. Brown the chops for about 4 minutes on each side. Add the wine. When it has reduced completely, turn the chops again and cook for another 2–3 minutes. Serve.

. . . .

Cristina Cuomo's Roasted Chicken with Root Vegetables

SERVES 4–6

Cristina likes to make this dish on autumn weekends when she is with her family in the Hamptons.

    15 small fresh figs
    1 x 1.75kg organic free-range chicken
    2 tablespoons olive oil
    Schwartz Chicken Seasoning
    2 tablespoons chopped fresh rosemary
    1.75kg mixed root vegetables, including 3 beetroots, 1 sweet

potato, 2 parsnips, several Brussels sprouts, and 5–10 shallots, all cubed.

3 cloves garlic

Preheat the oven to 200°C/gas mark 6.

Trim the ends off the figs and stuff as many into the cavity of the chicken as will fit. Set aside any extras.

Rub the chicken with the olive oil, seasoning, and rosemary. Place the chicken in a roasting dish and arrange the vegetables and garlic around it. Roast for 30 minutes, then turn the oven down to 190°C/gas mark 5. If you have set aside any figs, add them to the vegetables now.

Check the chicken after another 20 minutes. It is done when you make a small incision behind a leg and the juice runs clear. The total cooking time shouldn't be more than 1 hour.

. . . .

Rosemary-Roasted Trout

SERVES 4

I love to make this trout when I have company. Normally I would serve a trout per person, but in the name of portion control, here I allow one trout for two people.

salt and freshly ground black pepper

2 x 500g whole trout, cleaned, heads and tails left on

1 tablespoon finely chopped flat-leaf parsley

4 sprigs rosemary, leaves stripped and finely chopped

½ tablespoon finely chopped garlic, plus 3 cloves

2 tablespoons extra-virgin olive oil

juice of ½ lemon, plus 1 lemon cut into wedges

60ml white wine

Preheat the oven to 220°C/gas mark 7.

Salt and pepper the cavities of the trout. Mix the parsley,

rosemary, and chopped garlic. Rub the mixture into the flesh of the fish (not on the scale side).

Place the olive oil and garlic cloves in a roasting dish and add the trout, turning them once to coat both sides in the oil. Bake the fish for 15 minutes. The trout goes from rare to well-done in a matter of minutes. To see if it is the consistency you prefer, after 15 minutes cut a small slit near the spine of the fish. If it is done to your liking, remove the fish from the oven and douse with the lemon juice and white wine. If it needs a little more time, continue baking for another 3–8 minutes. Remove the trout from the oven.

To debone the trout, you need to start by cutting off the head with a sharp knife. Then pick up the fish by the tail and insert a fork into the meat of the fish. Gently pull up on the tail as you use the fork to hold down the meat. You will be inching toward the head of the fish (or where the head was before you removed it). Flip the fish over so the spine is now facing you. Hold the tail again as you insert the fork on the underside. Pull up on the tail as you use the fork to ease the meat off the bone. Discard the bones, transfer the meat to a plate, and serve with a wedge of lemon.

. . . .

Tom Colicchio's Poached Sea Bass with Roasted Tomato Vinaigrette and Fennel Salad

SERVES 4

This is a wonderful dinner party dish. I like it in winter when fennel is at its most aromatic.

Roasted Tomatoes
   10 ripe tomatoes, cut in half lengthwise and cores removed
   1 large head garlic, divided into unpeeled cloves

60ml extra-virgin olive oil

salt and freshly ground black pepper

4 sprigs fresh thyme

Vinaigrette

2 roasted tomato halves

60ml reserved roasted tomato juice, warm

2 tablespoons red wine vinegar

salt and freshly ground black pepper

125ml extra-virgin olive oil

Salad

1 small bulb fennel, cored and very thinly sliced

4 tablespoons mixed fresh herbs (such as tarragon, basil, chervil, dill, and parsley)

1 tablespoon extra-virgin olive oil

salt and freshly ground black pepper

Sea Bass

1 onion, chopped

1 carrot, peeled and sliced

1 stalk celery, sliced

1 head garlic, halved horizontally

3 sprigs parsley

3 sprigs thyme

1 bay leaf

10 peppercorns

2 teaspoons fennel seeds

1 teaspoon coriander seeds

225ml dry white wine

2 tablespoons salt

freshly ground pepper

4 sea bass fillets

Making the Tomatoes

Preheat the oven to 180°C/gas mark 4.

Place the tomato halves, garlic, and olive oil in a large bowl, season with salt and pepper, and mix gently. Line two large rimmed baking sheets with baking parchment or aluminium foil. Place the tomato halves on the baking sheets, cut side down, then pour any olive oil left in the bowl over them. Divide the garlic and thyme between the baking sheets and bake for about 20 minutes, until the tomato skins loosen. Remove and discard the skins. Pour any juice that has accumulated into a bowl and reserve.

Return the tomatoes to the oven and reduce the temperature to 140°C/gas mark 1. Continue roasting, periodically pouring off and reserving the juice, for 3–4 hours, until the tomatoes are slightly shrunken and appear cooked and concentrated but not yet dry.

Remove the tomatoes from the oven and allow them to cool on the baking sheets. Discard the thyme and reserve the tomatoes and juice separately.

Making the Vinaigrette

Combine the roasted tomatoes, reserved tomato juice, vinegar, salt, and pepper in a blender or food processor and puree. With the machine running, slowly add the olive oil and process until emulsified, then set aside.

Making the Salad

Combine the fennel and herbs in a small bowl. Dress with the olive oil, salt and pepper, and mix well.

Making the Sea Bass

Preheat the oven to 180°C/gas mark 4.

Make the vegetables and herbs into a bouquet garni and bring them to the boil in a pot. Lower the heat and simmer uncovered for 20–30 minutes. Strain, then pour the liquid back into the saucepan, add the wine, salt, and pepper, and place the sea bass skin side up. The liquid should not cover the skin.

Bake in the oven for 8 minutes, until the skin is crisp and the fish is tender. Remove from the oven and saucepan. To serve, divide the vinaigrette among four plates, arrange the sea bass over the vinaigrette, and top with the fennel salad.

. . . .

Eric Ripert's Grilled Salmon and Herb Salad with Toasted Sesame Seeds and Ponzu Vinaigrette

SERVES 4

I love how Eric has integrated South East Asian flavours into his menu. This dish reminds me of Thailand.

- 2 tablespoons soy sauce
- 2 tablespoons mirin (similar to sake)
- 3 tablespoons rice wine vinegar
- 2 tablespoons yuzu juice (This is almost impossible to find fresh in the United Kingdom. You can order bottled yuzu juice online.)
- 2 tablespoons lime juice
- fine sea salt and freshly ground pepper
- 60ml olive oil
- 60ml rapeseed oil, plus 1 tablespoon
- 700g salmon fillet, skin off and bones out
- 100g baby lettuce leaves
- 3–4 sprigs basil, leaves picked and torn
- 2 tablespoons mint leaves, torn
- 2 tablespoons coriander leaves, torn
- 1 tablespoon toasted sesame seeds

Preheat the grill. While it is heating, make the vinaigrette. In a small bowl, whisk together the soy sauce, mirin, rice wine vinegar, yuzu juice, and lime juice. Season to taste with salt and pepper; whisking constantly, slowly drizzle in the olive oil and the 60ml of rapeseed oil. The vinaigrette can be made ahead and stored up to two days in the refrigerator.

When the grill is ready, season the salmon fillet generously and evenly with the salt and pepper. Drizzle the 1 tablespoon of rapeseed oil over the salmon and sear it for 5–6 minutes on each side for medium-rare to medium. Remove the salmon from the grill and leave to stand on a cutting board.

Combine the baby lettuce with the herbs in a bowl. Flake the grilled salmon and place it in the bowl with the lettuce and herbs. Season the salad to taste with the salt and pepper and gently toss with 4 tablespoons of the vinaigrette.

Divide the salad onto four plates, sprinkle the toasted sesame seeds over the salad, and drizzle more of the vinaigrette around the salad. Serve immediately.

. . . .

Lidia Bastianich's Pan-Fried Chicken Breasts *Aglio e Olio*

SERVES 6

This dish should take less than 15 minutes to make, says Lidia.

6 chicken breast halves, skinless and boneless, about 900g total

¾ teaspoon salt, plus more as needed

75g flour

4 tablespoons extra-virgin olive oil

2 tablespoons butter

8 or more big cloves garlic, sliced

¼ teaspoon hot dried chilli flakes

3 tablespoons tiny capers in brine, drained

2 tablespoons red wine vinegar

225ml chicken or vegetable stock

1 tablespoon fine dry breadcrumbs
3 tablespoons chopped fresh flat-leaf parsley

With a paring knife, trim the chicken breast halves of all bits of fat, skin, and connective tissue. Do not cut off the tenders—the small loose flaps of muscle on the underside of each half—but flatten them firmly against the larger piece, to form a neat oval.

Sprinkle both sides of the breasts with about ½ teaspoon of the salt. Spread the flour on a piece of greaseproof paper and press and toss each breast in it to coat lightly on all surfaces; shake off excess.

Heat 2 tablespoons of the oil and all of the butter in the pan over a medium flame. When the butter is almost completely melted, lay the breasts in the pan with space between them. Let them cook in place, without moving them, until they're sizzling. After 2 minutes or so, lift the first breast you put in the pan and check the underside. You want it to be lightly tinged with brown (not pale, but not brown all over, either). Cook longer, if necessary, and then turn all of the breasts over when they've just begun to colour.

Quickly scatter all of the garlic slices into the spaces between the chicken, turn the heat up slightly, shake the pan, and stir the slices around in the hot fat so they separate. After 1 minute or a bit more, when the garlic has begun to sizzle, sprinkle the chilli flakes in a hot spot; toast for 1 minute; then spill the capers in several hot spots around the pan. Give the frying pan a few good shakes to distribute the seasonings and to make the hot juices run all around the breasts.

Raise the heat another notch. When everything's sizzling hard, pour the red wine vinegar into the open spaces and shake the pan to spread it. Let the vinegar sizzle and reduce for 30 seconds or so, then pour in the stock.

Cook at full blast now, quickly bringing the liquid to the boil. As it cooks, drizzle the remaining 2 tablespoons of oil all around the pan and sprinkle on the other ¼ teaspoon of salt. Let the sauce bubble and reduce for a couple of minutes as you shake the frying pan frequently, then sprinkle the bread-crumbs into the sauce (not on the chicken) and stir and shake. In 1–2 minutes, the crumbs will thicken the sauce visibly. Shake the frying pan until the sauce has the consistency you like. Turn off the heat, scatter the parsley over everything, and shake the frying pan again.

Serve right away. I usually bring the pan to the table and serve family-style. For a more formal presentation, spoon a pool of sauce onto a warm dinner plate, place a breast half on top, and moisten with a bit more sauce. Serve with vegetables.

. . . .

Mussels in Sake

SERVES 4

Mussels in white wine is a staple in French restaurants. I put an Asian spin on it by converting Gallic ingredients into more Eastern ones.

    1 tablespoon rapeseed
    25g chopped spring onions
    225ml sake
    1 clove garlic
    3 small red chillies with seeds, sliced thinly into rounds
    salt to taste
    1kg mussels
    3 tablespoons chopped coriander
    soy sauce to taste, optional

Place the rapeseed oil and spring onions in a large pot and sauté over a medium flame for 5 minutes. Add the sake, garlic, and chillies, boil, and reduce by half. Add the salt and mussels and cover. Cook for 10 minutes until the mussels open. Remove from the heat and sprinkle with the coriander. Stir. Transfer the mussels to a large serving bowl. If you like, you can mix in a spoonful of soy sauce.

. . . .

SIDE DISHES, SALADS, AND VEGETABLES
Chopped Salad Niçoise
SERVES 2

I started making this for Cesare when he was on a diet a few years ago. It remains a favourite whether we're weight-watching or not.

500g steamed asparagus, cut into 1-inch lengths

10 black olives

2 hard-boiled eggs, quartered

20 cherry tomatoes, halved

4 x 1-inch boiled potatoes, diced

125g oil-packed tuna, drained

2 tablespoons vinaigrette (see recipe on page 249)

200g mixed salad leaves

4 anchovy fillets

Place the first seven ingredients in a large bowl. Drizzle with the vinaigrette and toss gently. Divide the mixed salad leaves between two plates. Spoon the salad on top and garnish with the anchovies. Serve.

. . . .

Rocket and Chestnut Mushroom Salad
SERVES 2

This is another recipe from Cesare. He uses a few more ingredients, but this pared-down version is quicker and just as tasty.

1 tablespoon olive oil

4 teaspoons freshly squeezed lemon juice

2 teaspoons chopped flat-leaf parsley

salt and freshly ground black pepper

150g sliced chestnut mushrooms (button mushrooms will work if you can't find chestnut)

100g rocket

3 tablespoons shaved parmesan cheese

In a small bowl, whisk together the olive oil, lemon juice, parsley, salt, and pepper.

Place the mushrooms in a large bowl. Pour the dressing on top and toss to coat. Divide the rocket onto two plates. Spoon half of the mushroom mixture on top. Sprinkle the shaved parmesan on top and serve.

. . . .

Sautéed Spinach (or Swiss Chard)

SERVES 2

Follow the same directions to make sautéed Swiss chard.

500g fresh spinach, leaves torn into bite-size pieces

2 teaspoons olive oil

1 clove garlic, sliced

salt and freshly ground black pepper

After the spinach has been rinsed under running water, place it in a large pot with water still clinging to the leaves. Cover and cook for 7–8 minutes, stirring occasionally, until the leaves wilt. Drain in a colander.

Heat the oil in a medium frying pan and sauté the garlic until it starts to colour. Add the spinach and sauté briefly, about 2 minutes. Season with the salt and pepper and serve.

. . . .

Asparagus Salad

SERVES 4

This dish is best in May or June when asparagus is very tender. Use the thinnest stalks you can find.

1 tablespoon olive oil
1 tablespoon freshly squeezed lemon juice
salt and freshly ground black pepper
500g asparagus spears, sliced on the diagonal into 1-inch lengths
50g rocket
4 tablespoons shaved parmesan (for garnish)

In a small bowl, whisk together the oil, lemon juice, salt, and pepper. Place the asparagus in a bowl and toss with the dressing.

Divide the rocket onto four plates. Divide the asparagus into four amounts and spoon on top of the rocket. Garnish each salad with a tablespoon of parmesan. Serve.

. . . .

Spring Greens in Spicy Tomato Sauce

SERVES 6

I started making this dish with Tuscan kale, but that can be hard to find. Spring greens are even more substantial. For a main dish, serve this on top of pasta or any grain you like. For an appetizer, spoon 50gp on top of a crusty piece of toasted flat-leaf bread rubbed with garlic.

1kg spring greens, tough stems removed
1½ tablespoons olive oil
2 cloves garlic, sliced
½ teaspoon dried chilli flakes (or more, to taste)
2 x 400g cans plum tomatoes, juice reserved
salt

Fill a large pot with 2–3 inches of water. Add the spring greens, cover, and bring to a simmer. Cook about 20 minutes, stirring occasionally, until the greens are wilted. Drain and set aside.

While the spring greens are cooking, heat the olive oil in a large pot and sauté the garlic and chilli flakes until the garlic starts to colour. Crush the tomatoes with your hands and add them to the oil. Pour in the tomato juice from the can. Add the salt to taste and simmer for 20 minutes.

Add the spring greens and simmer another 5 minutes to blend the flavours. Adjust the seasoning and serve.

. . . .

Black Bean, Sweetcorn, and Tomato Salad

SERVES 6

This is a variation on a recipe by Julee Rosso and Sheila Lukins, the authors of the Silver Palate *cookbooks. I've been making it for years.*

> 500g canned black beans, rinsed
> 150g cooked fresh sweetcorn, sliced from the cob
> 200g chopped tomatoes
> 150g finely chopped green pepper
> 150g finely chopped red pepper
> 50g sliced spring onions
> 1 red chilli, seeds removed, finely chopped
> 3–4 tablespoons freshly squeezed lime juice
> zest of one lime
> 2 teaspoons cumin powder
> 2 teaspoons olive oil
> 2 tablespoons finely chopped coriander
> salt and freshly ground black pepper

Place the first seven ingredients in a large bowl and toss to mix well. In a small bowl, whisk together the lime juice, zest, cumin, olive oil, coriander, salt, and pepper. Pour over the vegetables and mix. Let the salad sit for 30 minutes before serving.

. . . .

Chicken Salad with Radicchio and Pine Nuts

SERVES 2

Cesare makes this dish with rabbit, and it's delicious, but in my opinion it's just as good with chicken or turkey. The sweetness of the meat and nuts is a great contrast to the bitterness of the radicchio.

225g cooked chicken breast, chopped

150g radicchio, torn into bite-size pieces

4 tablespoons toasted pine nuts

2 teaspoons olive oil

2 teaspoons water

2 teaspoons balsamic vinegar

2 teaspoons red wine vinegar

salt and freshly ground black pepper

In a large bowl, mix the chicken, radicchio, and pine nuts. In a small bowl, whisk the oil, water, vinegars, salt, and pepper. Pour over the salad and toss. Divide into two portions and serve.

. . . .

Roasted Radicchio

SERVES 4

I like this side dish with brown rice and chickpeas or on top of wholewheat pasta or quinoa.

2 large heads radicchio, cut into quarters, leaving part of core intact

1 tablespoon olive oil, plus 1 teaspoon

1 tablespoon red wine vinegar

1 tablespoon balsamic vinegar

1 tablespoon red wine

salt and freshly ground black pepper

Preheat the oven to 230°C/gas mark 8.

After the radicchio has been rinsed under running water, place it in a large bowl with water still clinging to the leaves and toss with the oil, vinegars, wine, salt, and pepper. Arrange the quarters, cut side up, on a baking sheet. Roast for 12 minutes. Remove from the oven and use tongs to turn each quarter over so the other side will brown. Return to the oven and roast another 8 minutes, until the quarters are wilted and tender.

. . . .

Tuscan Tuna Salad

SERVES 2

I never would have thought of combining canned tuna and beans, but it is a classic flat-leaf dish, usually served in seaside towns.

125g oil-packed tuna, drained
175g canned cannellini beans, drained and rinsed
2 tablespoons finely chopped red onion
200g chopped tomato
1 tablespoon chopped flat-leaf parsley
2 teaspoons olive oil
2 teaspoons freshly squeezed lemon juice
salt and freshly ground black pepper

Place the tuna, beans, red onion, tomato, and parsley in a bowl. Drizzle with the oil and lemon juice. Season with the salt and pepper to taste.

. . . .

Chicken Salad

SERVES 2

I poach chicken breast to make this recipe and freeze the stock to make other dishes, but you can also use leftover roasted chicken for the salad.

1 tablespoon mayonnaise
1 teaspoon Dijon mustard

1 teaspoon red wine vinegar
25g finely chopped celery
1 tablespoon finely chopped red onion
150g diced cooked chicken breast
200g mixed salad leaves

Combine the mayonnaise, mustard, and vinegar in a small bowl. Stir in the celery and red onion until well mixed. Add the chicken and mix to coat well.

Divide the lettuce onto two plates. Spoon the chicken salad on top and serve.

. . . .

Salmon Salad

SERVES 2

This recipe reminds me of my mom, who loved canned salmon. It's comfort food for me.

225g canned salmon, drained
25g finely chopped celery
1 tablespoon finely chopped red onion
2 teaspoons finely chopped dill
1 tablespoon mayonnaise
salt and freshly ground black pepper
mixed salad leaves

Place the salmon in a bowl and flake. Add the celery, red onion, and dill. Stir in the mayonnaise and season with the salt and pepper. Serve on top of salad leaves.

. . . .

Roasted Root Vegetables

SERVES 4–5

This is a staple on my dinner table. The squash and onions cara-melize, which gives the dish a sweet kick. You can roast almost any vegetable following the same steps described here. I also prepare cauliflower, Brussels sprouts, broccoli, and asparagus this way. You will have to adjust the cooking time, depending on the vegetable. Cauliflower and broccoli take about 20 minutes; asparagus needs about 10. Turn all vegetables at least once during cooking.

    400g 1-inch cubes butternut squash
    300g 1-inch cubes parsnips
    300g 1-inch cubes red onion
    300g 1-inch cubes turnips
    2–3 tablespoons olive oil
    1 tablespoon water (if needed)
    1 teaspoon dried chilli flakes (or to taste)
    1–2 teaspoons salt

Preheat the oven to 220°C/gas mark 7.

Place the vegetables in a large bowl and drizzle with the olive oil. Use your hands to mix the vegetables and oil together so that the vegetables are well-coated. If they feel dry, add the water and mix again. Mix in the chilli flakes and salt.

Spread the vegetables on a non-stick baking sheet and place it in the oven. After 20 minutes, remove the vegetables from the oven and turn, using a spatula. Return to the oven for another 20 minutes. Remove and serve.

Roasted Butternut Squash

SERVES 3–4

Roasted butternut squash is almost like a dessert.

    800g 1-inch cubes butternut squash
    150g 1-inch cubes red onion (optional)
    4 teaspoons olive oil
    1 teaspoon dried chilli flakes (or to taste)
    1–2 teaspoons salt

Preheat the oven to 220°C/gas mark 7.

Place the vegetables in a large bowl and toss well. Drizzle the olive oil and toss again. Add the chilli flakes over the vegetables and salt. Toss, then spread the vegetables on a non-stick baking sheet. Roast 10 to 15 minutes until the edges start to brown. Stir and return to the oven for another 5 to 10 minutes, or until the squash is tender and caramelized. Remove and serve.

. . . .

Tomato Bruschetta

SERVES 2

In summer, when tomatoes are at their peak, I double this recipe and make a meal of it, with some olives and a glass of wine.

200g diced tomato

1 tablespoon finely chopped spring onions

1 tablespoon finely chopped basil

2 teaspoons olive oil

2 teaspoons red wine vinegar

salt and freshly ground black pepper

1 clove garlic

2 thin slices toasted crusty bread

Place the tomatoes, spring onions, and basil in a bowl and toss. In a separate bowl, whisk the oil, vinegar, salt, and pepper. Cut the garlic clove in half and rub the cut side over the toast. Spoon the tomato mixture over the bread and serve.

. . . .

Bruschetta with Beans

SERVES 4

Beans are one the healthiest foods you can eat. They're full of protein and fibre. I like them cooked until they are very tender.

    1 tablespoon olive oil
    2 teaspoons red wine vinegar
    2 teaspoons chopped parsley
    salt and freshly ground black pepper
    100g cooked cannellini beans
    50g chopped tomatoes
    2 tablespoons sliced spring onions
    4 slices toasted crusty bread

In a small bowl, whisk together the oil, vinegar, parsley, salt, and pepper. In a separate bowl, toss the beans, tomatoes, and spring onions. Pour the dressing over the bean mixture and mix. Spoon a quarter of the bruschetta mixture onto each piece of toast and serve.

. . . .

Caesar Salad

SERVES 2

This recipe has a little more kick but a lot fewer calories than the traditional one. I left out the raw egg. You don't need it, and for safety reasons, why risk it? If you want, you can add a little hard-boiled egg to the dressing.

    1 clove garlic
    200g romaine lettuce, torn into bite-size pieces
    ½ teaspoon salt
    2 anchovy fillets, oil rinsed off
    2 tablespoons freshly squeezed lemon juice
    1 tablespoon Worcestershire sauce
    2 teaspoons olive oil
    2 tablespoons grated parmesan cheese
    freshly ground black pepper
    4 tablespoons croutons (for garnish)

Cut the garlic clove in half and rub the cut side on the inside of a salad bowl. Add the lettuce and set aside.

Place the garlic clove in a mortar. Add the salt and use the pestle to grind the two into a paste. Add the anchovies and continue to grind until the anchovies are mixed well with the garlic. Transfer the paste to a small mixing bowl. Stir in the lemon juice and Worcestershire sauce and drizzle in the olive oil, then add the parmesan cheese. Spoon over the romaine and toss well. Adjust the seasoning, garnish with the croutons, and serve.

. . . .

Marcus Samuelsson's Tomato-Watermelon Salad with Almond Vinaigrette

SERVES 6

I have been following Marcus Samuelsson's career for years and even wrote a book proposal with him before he was a super chef. The flavours in this salad are unexpected and delicious. It's so satisfying on a hot summer afternoon.

- 2 tablespoons flaked almonds
- 4 garlic cloves, thinly sliced
- 2 teaspoons harissa*
- 3 tablespoons extra-virgin olive oil
- 1 tablespoon sherry vinegar
- juice of 1 lime
- 2 shallots, thinly sliced
- 150g cubed watermelon (¾-inch cubes)
- 1 red chilli, seeds and ribs removed, thinly sliced
- 2 tablespoons torn parsley leaves
- 2 tablespoons torn mint leaves
- 1 tablespoon capers
- ½ teaspoon salt
- freshly ground black pepper
- 3 red tomatoes, roughly chopped (about 200g)
- 3 yellow tomatoes, roughly chopped (about 200g)
- 75g crumbled goat's cheese

To make the vinaigrette, combine the almonds, garlic, and harissa in a small pan over a medium flame and sauté for 3 minutes. Remove from the heat.

Combine the olive oil, vinegar, lime juice, and shallots in a small bowl. Whisk in the almond-harissa mixture.

Toss the watermelon, chilli, parsley, mint, and capers in a large bowl. Season with the salt and a few grindings of pepper. Add the tomatoes and vinaigrette and toss to combine. Garnish with the goat's cheese and serve immediately.

*Harissa, the fiery red chilli paste from Tunisia, is typically added to couscous, soups, and stews, but I like to use it as a super-spicy condiment as well. Premade harissa can be found in specialist shops, most supermarkets, or online.

. . . .

Lentil Salad

SERVES 6

I add even more mustard than this recipe calls for because I like the extra kick.

175g green lentils
100g finely chopped red onion
24 pitted green and black olives, chopped
3 tablespoons chopped parsley
1–2 tablespoons Dijon mustard
2 tablespoons red wine vinegar
1 tablespoon olive oil
2 teaspoons salt
freshly ground black pepper

Bring the lentils to the boil in 1 litre of water in a large saucepan. Lower the heat and simmer about 40 minutes, until the lentils are tender. Drain and set aside.

Combine the onion, olives, and parsley in a bowl. In a separate bowl, whisk together the mustard and vinegar until well blended. Then whisk in the olive oil and beat until emul-sified. Add the salt and pepper.

Pour half of the dressing over the onion mixture and combine. Gently stir in the lentils and the remaining dressing.

· ·

Avocado and Grapefruit Salad with Citrus Dressing

SERVES 4

Dee Dee DeBartlo, one of my journal keepers, gave me this recipe. I love the grapefruit and avocado together.

Dressing
  1 tablespoon grapefruit or orange juice
  1 tablespoon freshly squeezed lemon juice
  2 tablespoons olive oil
  ¼ teaspoon salt
  freshly ground black pepper

Salad
  2 avocados, halved, pitted, peeled, and thinly sliced
  1 large pink grapefruit, peeled with pith removed, segments
    cut from between membranes
  300g Little Gem or loose-leaf lettuce

In a small bowl, whisk together the citrus juices, olive oil, salt, and pepper. Place the avocado slices and grapefruit sections in a bowl. Pour the dressing over and toss gently.

Arrange the lettuce on four salad plates. Divide the avocado and grapefruit evenly and spoon onto the lettuce. Serve.

· ·

Spinach Salad with Artichokes and Lemon Dressing

SERVES 4

Another Dee Dee DeBartlo special, but I reduced the amount of olive oil. You can get away with even less.

Dressing
3 tablespoons freshly squeezed lemon juice
2 tablespoons olive oil
pinch salt
freshly ground black pepper

Salad
125g baby spinach
8–10 canned artichoke hearts, quartered
1 red pepper, sliced into ¼-inch strips
3 hard-boiled eggs, sliced into quarters lengthwise
50g chopped kalamata olives

In a small bowl, whisk together the dressing ingredients.

Place the salad components in a large bowl and drizzle with the dressing. Toss to mix well and divide onto four plates. Serve.

. . . .

Roasted Kale Crisps

SERVES 2

After an estate agent I interviewed mentioned these crisps, I went straight home and made a batch. I'm totally addicted to them.

1 bag kale
1 tablespoon olive oil
salt

Preheat the oven to 200°C/gas mark 6.

To strip the curly part of the kale leaf from the thick stem, you can use either scissors or your fingers. Discard the stems and tear the leaves into bite-size pieces. Place the leaves in a large bowl and drizzle the oil over them. Salt and toss well. Spread the leaves on a baking sheet lined with baking parchment. Bake 10–15 minutes, until the edges are just turning brown.

. . . .

Mario Batali's Misticanza

SERVES 6

In Greek, fennel, the main ingredient here, means to grow thin, or so I've read. Perhaps that's why it's popular with dieters. I just like the flavour. Plus, anything Mario makes tastes good to me

Vinaigrette (makes 175ml)

60ml freshly squeezed lemon juice

1 teaspoon lemon marmalade or a generous pinch of grated lemon zest

125ml extra-virgin olive oil, preferably Tuscan

Salad

1 small fennel bulb, trimmed

225g radishes, trimmed

240g (3 medium bags) rocket, trimmed

Maldon or other sea salt flakes and coarsely ground black pepper

Whisk together the lemon juice, marmalade, and olive oil in a small bowl. The vinaigrette can be refrigerated for up to three days.

Using a vegetable slicer, thinly shave the fennel. Transfer to a medium bowl. Thinly shave the radishes and add to the bowl. Add the rocket and toss gently. Drizzle with half the vinaigrette, tossing gently. Season with the salt and pepper and serve with the remaining vinaigrette on the side.

. . . .

SALAD DRESSINGS, DIPS, AND SPREADS

Asian-Style Dressing for Green Beans or Salad Leaves

MAKES ABOUT 175ml DRESSING, OR ABOUT 6 SERVINGS

I started making this dressing for green beans, but now I use it on everything from asparagus to salads. It's even nice on apples.

> 60ml white wine vinegar
> 1 tablespoon soy sauce
> 2 teaspoons sesame oil
> 2 tablespoons sliced spring onions
> salt and freshly ground black pepper
> 2 tablespoons toasted sesame seeds

Place the vinegar, soy sauce, sesame oil, spring onions, salt, and pepper in a small jar that closes tightly. Cover and shake well, until emulsified. Stir in seeds. This will keep for a few days in the refrigerator.

. . . .

Vinaigrette

SERVES 1

Traditional vinaigrettes tend to use twice as much oil as vinegar, with a shot of mustard for a little kick. I reverse the proportions. It makes a strong, flavourful dressing, so you won't need a lot.

> 1 small clove garlic, finely chopped
> 60ml vinegar
> salt and freshly ground black pepper
> 2 tablespoons Dijon mustard
> 1 tablespoon olive oil

Whisk together the garlic, vinegar, salt, pepper, and mustard in a small bowl. Continue whisking as you drizzle in the oil. Store the dressing in a jar and shake well before reusing. This will keep for a week in the refrigerator.

. . . .

Honey-Dijon Dressing

MAKES 175ml

Paula Chin, a foodie friend of mine and Family Circle *editor, swears by this dressing.*

- 1 tablespoon Dijon mustard
- 3 tablespoons balsamic vinegar
- 1½ teaspoons soy sauce
- 2 tablespoons honey
- 3 tablespoons plain yogurt
- 3 tablespoons olive oil
- salt and pepper to taste

Whisk together the mustard and vinegar, then whisk in the remaining ingredients until smooth.

. . . .

Erika's Olive Tapenade

MAKES ABOUT 750g

Erika, who is part Armenian, got this recipe from her sister. She spreads it on toasted baguette slices, pitta, or crackers, and she even adds it to scrambled eggs and soups. (All amounts are approximate, to taste.)

- 700g pitted kalamata olives in oil-based marinade
- 700g pitted kalamata olives in vinegar-based marinade
- 2–3 tablespoons freshly squeezed lemon juice
- 3–4 cloves garlic
- 1–2 teaspoons capers

2–3 anchovy fillets

125ml olive oil

Rinse the olives in cold water to remove any oil or brine.

In batches, combine all ingredients except the oil in a food processor; drizzle the oil through the pour spout. Blend into a rough paste—no chunks, but not too gummy.

. . . .

Lemony Hummus
MAKES ABOUT 600g

A Lebanese friend gave me this recipe in 1982. I've been using it ever since.

2 x 400g cans chickpeas, drained and rinsed

2 tablespoons water

2 small cloves garlic

175g tahini (sesame paste)

60ml freshly squeezed lemon juice

salt and freshly ground black pepper

paprika

Put the chickpeas, water, and garlic in a food processor and blend until smooth. Transfer to a bowl. Thin the tahini with the lemon juice and stir into the pureed chickpeas. Add the salt and pepper to taste. Sprinkle with the paprika and serve.

Spinach Dip
MAKES ABOUT 600g

My friend Paula adapted this recipe from Ladies Home Journal. *I switched the yogurt from low-fat (which she suggests) to full-fat yogurt.*

1 tablespoon olive oil

150g chopped onion

2 teaspoons finely chopped garlic

½ teaspoon cumin

275g frozen chopped spinach, thawed

3 tablespoons pine nuts, lightly toasted

½ teaspoon salt (or more, to taste)

freshly ground black pepper

125g plain yogurt

Heat the oil and sauté the onions on a medium-low flame for 10 minutes, or until transluscent. Add the garlic and cumin and sauté 5 minutes more. In the meantime, take the spinach by handfuls, squeeze out the excess liquid, and transfer to the food processor. Add the onions, pine nuts, salt, pepper, and yogurt. Pulse until well blended.

· ·

Anchovy Dip

MAKES ABOUT 500g

I first had this dip in Piedmont in Italy, where it is a local speciality. Locals serve it warm with assorted crudités. I like it best with broccoli. It is very intense, so just a tablespoon will do.

225ml olive oil

3 cloves garlic

125ml white wine

75g anchovy fillets, drained

225ml water

salt and freshly ground black pepper

steamed broccoli florets

Heat the olive oil in a medium saucepan and gently simmer the garlic over a medium-low flame for 6–7 minutes. Don't let the oil come to the boil. Add the wine and continue cooking for 5 minutes. Add the anchovies and water and, stirring occasionally, cook another 30 minutes, or until the anchovies have dissolved. Add the salt and pepper to taste. Remove from heat and serve with broccoli.

. . . .

DESSERTS

Chocolate Pudding

SERVES 8

This recipe is a variation of one a friend of mine found on About.com. For fewer calories you can use skimmed milk. It's so rich, all you need is a demitasse—and a baby spoon, so the pudding lasts longer.

> 50g white sugar
> 50g demerara sugar
> 50g cocoa powder
> 75g cornflour
> 50g dark chocolate chips
> 500ml milk
> 3–4 tablespoons brewed espresso
> 2 tablespoons brandy

Place the sugars, cocoa powder, cornflour, and chocolate chips in a small saucepan. Add the milk and bring to a low boil over a medium flame, stirring constantly. Reduce heat and stir until thickened. Remove from the heat. Stir in the espresso and brandy. Pour into eight 50ml demitasse cups. Serve warm.

. . . .

Chocolate Peanut Butter Pudding

SERVES 2

This is an alternative to chocolate pudding. My friend Janet stumbled onto this recipe while experimenting with frozen drinks. She put some leftover smoothie in the refrigerator, and the next day discovered pudding. She also makes her own chocolate sauce using cocoa powder, soya milk, and honey, but bottled chocolate sauce is fine, too.

1 banana
2 tablespoons peanut butter
3 tablespoons chocolate syrup
175ml milk or soya milk

Place all the ingredients in a blender and combine until smooth. Pour into two ramekins and chill overnight in the refrigerator.

. . . .

Oat Cookies

MAKES 36 COOKIES

These are adapted from Theresa Passarelli, who herself adapted the recipe from EatingWell. *They're dense and delicious.*

200g brown sugar
175g low-fat yogurt
1 large egg white, lightly beaten
2 tablespoons vegetable oil
2 tablespoons brandy
100g dessicated coconut
100g chocolate chips
175g rolled oats
150g sifted plain flour
100g ground flaxseeds
1 teaspoon ground cinnamon
½ teaspoon salt

Preheat the oven to 180°C/gas mark 4.

Place the brown sugar, yogurt, egg white, oil, and brandy in a large bowl and mix well. Stir in the dessicated coconut and the chocolate chips. Stir in the oats. Stir in the flour, flaxseeds, cinnamon, and salt.

Drop the mixture by the tablespoon on a non-stick baking sheet or a baking sheet lined with parchment. Flatten slightly and space about an inch apart. Bake 12–15 minutes, until lightly browned. Transfer the cookies to a wire rack and cool.

. . . .

Sources

1. Forget the French

Barbaro, Michael. "Mayor Doesn't Always Live by His Health Rules." *New York Times*, September 22, 2009.

Chan, Sewell. "Bronx's Weight Is Up, and Manhattan's Is Down." *New York Times*, July 21, 2009.

Christakis, Nicholas, and James Fowler. "The Spread of Obesity in a Large Social Network over 32 Years." *New England Journal of Medicine*, 357, no. 4 (July 26, 2007): 370–379. http://www.nejm.org/doi/full/10.1056/NEJMsa066082#t=articleTop.

Citizens Committee for New York City. "Speak Out New York: Neighborhood Quality of Life Survey Report." April 7, 2008. www.citizensnyc.org.

"New York City Passes Trans Fat Ban." MSNBC News Services, December 5, 2006.

2. A Manhattan State of Mind

"The Biggest Retailer in the World Covers an Area Larger Than Manhattan." *Good*, November/December 2007.

Wansink, Brian. *Mindless Eating: Why We Eat More Than We Think*. New York: Bantam Books, 2006.

3. Dark Chocolate, Almonds, and Discipline

Bollinger, Bryan, Phillip Leslie, and Alan Sorensen. "Calorie Postings in Chain Restaurants." January 2010. www.stanford.edu/~pleslie/calories.pdf.

"City Limits Guide to Food Access in NYC." 2004. http://www.citylimits.org.

Cohen, Yael. "Fashion Week Food Diaries." *New York*, February 18, 2007.

Elbel, Brian, Rogan Kersh, Victoria L. Brescoll, and L. Beth Dixon. "Calorie Labeling and Food Choices: A First Look at the Effects on Low-Income People in New York City." *Health Affairs*, October 2009. http://content. healthaffairs.org/content/early/2009/10/06/hlthaff.28.6.w1110.full. pdf+html. Published online before print October 2009, doi: 10.1377/ hlthaff.28.6.w1110 *Health Aff October 2009*.

4. Grocery Love

Drewnowski, Adam. "Obesity and the Food Environment: Dietary Energy Density and Diet Costs." *American Journal of Preventive Medicine* 27, no. 3 (October 2004): 154–162.

"Greenmarket Map 2011," http://www.grownyc.org.

U.S. Department of Agriculture. "Your Food Environment Atlas." 2006. http://maps.ers.usda.gov/FoodAtlas/.

Wang, May C., Soowon Kim, Alma A. Gonzalez, Kara E. MacLeod, and Marilyn A. Winkleby. "Socioeconomic and Food-Related Physical Characteristics of the Neighbourhood Environment Are Associated with Body Mass Index." *Journal of Epidemiology and Community Health* 61, no. 6: 491–498.

5. Walk the Walk, Talk the Talk

Black, Jennifer L., and James Macinko. "The Changing Distribution and Determinants of Obesity in the Neighborhoods of New York City, 2003–2007." *American Journal of Epidemiology* 171, no. 7 (February 19, 2010): 765–775.

Colletti, Jaclyn, and Maria Masters. "America's Fattest Cities." *Men's Health*, 2010. http://www.menshealth.com/fattestcities2010/.

Dominus, Susan. "Getting Slim Just by Riding the Subway." *New York Times*, July 17, 2010.

MacDonald, John M., Robert J. Stokes, Deborah A. Cohen, Aaron Kofner, and Greg K. Ridgeway. "The Effect of Light Rail Transit on Body Mass Index and Physical Activity." *American Journal of Preventative Medicine* 39, no. 2 (August 2010): 105–112.

Oswald, Andrew, and Stephen Wu. "Research Finds the Happiest US States Match a Million Americans' Own Happiness States." *Science*, December 17, 2009.

RAND Corporation, Center for Population Health and Health Disparities. "Park Use and Physical Activity in a Sample of Public Parks in the City of Los Angeles." 2006. http://www.rand.org/pubs/technical_reports/TR357.html.

Sperling's Best Places. "New Study Pulls the Blanket off America's Best and Worst Cities for Sleep." This study was done in partnership with Sanofi-Aventis, the makers of Ambien, a prescription sleep medication. http://bestplaces.net/docs/studies/ambiensleep.aspx.

Thompson, Clive. "Why New Yorkers Last Longer." *New York*, August 13, 2007.

"2009 Fittest/Fattest Cities." *Men's Health*. http://www.mensfitness.com/outdoors/travel-destinations/2009-fittest-fattest-cities.

7. White Truffle Risotto and Other Dilemmas

Berman, Mark, and Risa Lavizzo-Mourey. "Obesity Prevention in the Information Age: Caloric Information at the Point of Purchase." *Journal of the American Medical Association* 300(4) (2008): 433–435. http://jama.ama-assn.org/.

Brunstrom, J. M., and P. J. Rogers. "How Many Calories Are on Our Plate? Expected Fullness, Not Liking, Determines Meal-Size Selection." *Obesity* 17, no. 10 (October 2009): 1884–1890.

Chernev, Alexander. "The Dieter's Paradox." *Journal of Consumer Psychology* 21(2) (August 2010): 178–183.

Hurely, Jayne, and Bonnie Liebman "Extreme Eating 2010." *Nutrition Action Health Letter*, June 2010.

Levenstein, Harvey. *Revolution at the Table: The Transformation of the American Diet*. New York: Oxford University Press, 1988.

McColl, Karen. "The Fattening Truth about Restaurant Food." November 18, 2008. http://www.BMJ.com.

Mercola, Joseph. "Tricks Restaurants Use to Make You Eat More and Faster." May 18, 2010. http://www.lewrockwell.com.

Obbagy, J. E., M. D. Condrasky, L. S. Roe, J. L. Sharp, and B. J. Rolls. "Chefs' Opinions about Reducing the Calorie Content of Menu Items in Restaurants. *Obesity* 19, no. 2 (February 2011): 332–337.

Richardson, Whit. "Does Portland Have More Restaurants Per Capita than San Francisco?" August 18, 2009. http://www.mainebiz.biz.

Wansink, Brian. *Mindless Eating: Why We Eat More Than We Think*. New York: Bantam Books, 2006.

Wansink, B., and P. Chandon. "Meal Size, Not Body Size, Explains Errors in Estimating the Calorie Content of Meals." *Annals of Internal Medicine* 145, no. 5 (September 5, 2006): 326–332.

8. Okay, We Cheat

Horton, T. J., H. Drougas, A. Brachey, G. W. Reed, J. C. Peters, and J. O. Hill. "Fat and Carbohydrate Overfeeding in Humans: Different Effects on Energy Storage." *American Journal of Clinical Nutrition*, 62, no. 1 (1995): 19–29.

Mann, Traci. "Dieting Does Not Work." *American Psychologist*, April 2007.

Reisner, Rebecca. "The Diet Industry: A Big Fat Lie." *Bloomberg Businessweek*, January 2008.

Weyer, C., B. Vozarova, E. Ravussin, and P. A. Tataranni. "Changes in Energy Metabolism in Response to 48 H of Overfeeding and Fasting in Caucasians and Pima Indians." *International Journal of Obesity* 25, no. 5 (May 2001): 593–600.

Wolpert, Stuart. "Dieting Doesn't Work: UCLA Researchers Find That People Who Lose Weight Usually Gain It All Back—Plus Some." *UCLA Magazine*, April 4, 2007.

9. Expert Handling

Johnston, Laura. "Effectiveness of Registered Dietitian-Guided Weight Loss over the Phone and Internet." http://www.dietbattles.com.

Leppert, Phyllis, and Jeffrey Peipert. *Primary Care for Women*. New York: Lippincott Williams and Wilkens, 2004.

Myers, Anita M. *Program Evaluation for Exercise Leaders*. Champaigne, IL: Human Kinetics, 1999.

Raatz, Susan K. "Consulting a Registered Dietitian Aids Weight Loss." *Journal of the American Dietetic Association* 108 (January 2008): 110–113.

Weinberg, Robert, and Daniel Gould. *Foundations of Sport and Exercise Psychology*. 5th ed. Champaigne, IL: Human Kinetics, 2011.

10. Confident in the Kitchen

Harry Balzer. "Americans Are Eating at Home More; Microwave Usage Increases, but Not Cooking." NPD Group, Chicago, Illinois, November 12, 2009.

Cockcroft, Lucy. "A Home-Cooked Meal in 2008 Contains Half the Ingredients of a 1950s Dinner." *Telegraph* (London), July 8, 2008. http://www.telegraph.co.uk/news/uknews/2265774/A-home-cooked-meal-in-2008-contains-half-the-ingredients-of-a-1950s-dinner.html.

"New York City Food Lover's Guide," *Zagat's*, July 2009.

Pew Research Center. "Eating More; Enjoying Less." April 19, 2006. *pewresearch.org*.

U.S. Energy Information Administration. "Are We Really Becoming a Fast-Food Country?" 2001. http://205.254.135.24/emeu/recs/cookingtrends/cooking.html.

Index

Acknowledgements

Thank you first to all of the amazing and generous women who shared their stories, tips, and crazy habits with me. Without you, I'd have no book. Ditto for all of my diary keepers, who tracked their every bite, large and small, in service of creating the Manhattan Diet (I would list you by name, but I promised anonymity). Between Joanne Lipman, Amy Stevens, Hilary Stout, Bill Tonelli, Lauren Lipton, Nancy Farkas, Susie Adams, Janet Ungless, Shari Steinberg, Ruth Porat, and Dana Weinstein, I had the world's greatest cheerleading squad. You are all awesome. Thank you to Tom Weber, photographer supreme, and Kim Diamond, my nutritional guru. Thank you to Caitlin McNiff for networking so diligently on my behalf and to Dorothy Hamilton for listening, advising, and offering a helping hand. Thank you to Richard Pine for taking on this project and to Tom Miller for snapping it up. Thank you to my dad, Michael Daspin, for everything, and to my mom, Sara, for her guiding spirit. And most of all, thank you to my best eating and partner in all things foodie and otherwise, Cesare Casella. And thank you to Chen Casella, for just being your delicious self.